Breastfeeding with Confidence

Sue Cox

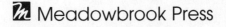

Meadowbrook Press

Distributed by Simon & Schuster
New York

Library of Congress Cataloging-in-Publication Data

Cox, Sue.
  Breastfeeding with confidence : a practical guide / Sue Cox.
    p. cm.
  Summary: "A practical, helpful guide to help you learn the art and method of breastfeeding"—
Provided by publisher.
  ISBN 0-88166-513-4 (Meadowbrook Press) ISBN 0-684-04005-0 (Simon & Schuster)
  1. Breastfeeding—Handbooks, manuals, etc. 2. Breastfeeding—Popular works. I. Title.
  RJ216.C693 2006
  649'.33—dc22
                    2006007014

Editorial Director: Christine Zuchora-Walske
Editor: Angela Wiechmann
Contributing Editors: Denise Fisher, Molly Pessl
Proofreader: Megan McGinnis
Production Manager: Paul Woods
Graphic Design Manager: Tamara Peterson
Cover Photo: Plush Studios
Interior Illustrations: Coral Tulloch
Index: Beverlee Day

© 2006 by Sue Cox. This book was originally published by Finch Publishing in Australia and New Zealand as *Breastfeeding with Confidence* based on the original manuscript titled *Breastfeeding I Can Do That.*

Illustration on page 3 modified from D. Ramsay (2005).

Every effort has been made to obtain permission to reproduce material from other sources. Where permission could not be obtained, the publisher welcomes hearing from the copyright holder(s) in order to acknowledge that copyright.

The contents of this book have been reviewed and checked for accuracy and appropriateness by professionals in the field of human lactation. However, the authors, editors, reviewers, and publisher disclaim all responsibility arising from any adverse effects or results that occur or might occur as a result of the inappropriate application of any of the information contained in this book. If you have a question or concern about any of the information in this book, consult your healthcare professional.

Published by Meadowbrook Press, 5451 Smetana Drive, Minnetonka, Minnesota 55343

www.meadowbrookpress.com

BOOK TRADE DISTRIBUTION by Simon and Schuster, a division of Simon and Schuster, Inc., 1230 Avenue of the Americas, New York, NY 10020

11 10 09 08 07 06   10 9 8 7 6 5 4 3 2 1

Printed in the United States of America

To Harry, who taught me, among other things, to believe in myself;
Brian and Christine, who are proof that positive parenting works;
Mary, with whom I learned the early skills of mothering;
and all the families I've had the privilege to work with.

Acknowledgments

My knowledge of breastfeeding has come from four sources. First, from my children, Brian and Christine, who gave me confidence when they thrived as babies—even though I worried whether I was feeding them enough. They taught me that there are no set rules for breastfeeding. As they grew from newborns to healthy, loving children and now adults, they confirmed my belief in the importance of breastfeeding.

Second, from the women I've had the privilege to talk to and learn from, whether they were new mothers, breastfeeding counselors, or the most experienced lactation consultants. You'll find letters from some of these women in this book. I contacted many of the mothers, and they're pleased that their stories have been included. (For the women I wasn't able to contact, I changed their names.) I thank all these women for their letters and the assistance they'll give to other mothers and babies.

Third, and most importantly, from my questioning nature, which made me ask "But why?" many times. The answers came from people in the lactation field, particularly Professor Peter Hartmann, whom I first heard speak in 1982. His presentation about human milk research gave me the basis to question hospital routines and the courage to convince people that the art of breastfeeding would be so much easier if it were based on biochemistry and physiology.

The fourth source was my own eyes. Every day I watch women breastfeed their babies, and this has helped me combine the art and the science. I thank Rebecca Glover for teaching me how to *see* instead of how to *watch*.

This book has evolved throughout the years. Many people have asked how I found the time and energy to write my original book, *Breastfeeding I Can Do That*, which I self-published in 1997. Obviously, my personal drive and commitment kept me going, but Harry, my husband, and Christine, my daughter, gave me the support I needed to focus on writing and be free of household responsibilities. My friends, colleagues, and clients also supported me and helped me believe this was an important book. A number of them, including Andrea Davey, Jo Gratten, Barbara Attrill, Maryanne Davis, Cynthia Turnbull, Bronwyn Hinchcliffe, Ruth Feegar, and Elisa and John McGuiness, reviewed the first draft. Denise Fisher's constructive criticism also had a profound effect on the manuscript, and Dr. Tom Hale's review of medications was invaluable. It was a privilege to work with Coral Tulloch, whose illustrations added an extra dimension to the first edition—and each edition after it. Her art makes this more than an educational tool. My thanks to Melinda and baby Holly, and Wendy and baby Isaac for being Coral's models and becoming part of this book.

Breastfeeding I Can Do That evolved into *Breastfeeding with Confidence* with Finch Publishing in 2004. The impetus came from my friend and colleague, Joy Heads, OAM, who introduced me to Dr. Howard Chilton (author of *Baby on Board*), who subsequently introduced me to Rex Finch and Finch Publishing. My son, Brian, patiently and expertly taught me some tech skills that were absolutely invaluable during the creation of the Finch edition.

Rex Finch's negotiations led to this latest evolution of *Breastfeeding with Confidence* with Meadowbrook Press. It has been a very rewarding experience and a great pleasure to work with the editorial and publicity staff at Meadowbrook Press, most particularly Angela Wiechmann, whose imaginative editing came from her extraordinary insight into relationships, parenting, and breastfeeding. I'm delighted that her relocation of information, incisive probing, and helpful suggestions have led to many important changes in this edition. Angie received valuable input from my colleagues and contributing editors Denise Fisher, IBCLC, and Molly Pessl, IBCLC. She also received great support from editorial director Christine Zuchora-Walske, proofreader Megan McGinnis, production manager Paul Woods, graphic design manager Tamara Peterson, and indexer Beverlee Day.

And finally, I give my eternal thanks and love to my husband, Harry, whose analytical probing completed the transformation of my original words into the polished final manuscripts in 1997, 2002, 2004, and now with this edition.

Contents

Foreword

Breastfeeding with Confidence is the most helpful basic book on breastfeeding I have ever read. Sue Cox is a pioneer in this field—she has been an Australian Breastfeeding Association (ABA) counselor for thirty years, an International Board Certified Lactation Consultant (IBCLC) since the first year the credential became available in 1985, and the ABA's first delegate to the International Board of Lactation Consultant Examiners (IBLCE). She's a well-known author who practices as an IBCLC and midwife in her native Hobart, Tasmania, Australia. Her renown propelled her into the presidency of the International Lactation Consultant Association (ILCA) for the 2005–6 term.

Breastfeeding with Confidence is the answer for women who are a bit daunted by the prospect of breastfeeding or who simply want clear, practical solutions to both common and uncommon problems. Although it doesn't wade through every possible solution to every possible problem, it does provide a wealth of recommended resources in case women have special concerns that aren't addressed in the book. Upbeat and cheerful, practical and positive, *Breastfeeding with Confidence* does indeed build confidence in women's ability to master what many expect to be a simple, natural process but so often is not.

—JoAnne W. Scott, MA, IBCLC,
Executive Director of IBLCE for twenty years

Introduction

Over the many years I've been supporting breastfeeding mothers, women frequently ask me what's the best way to learn how to breastfeed. I often say learning how to breastfeed is a lot like learning how to drive a car.

Remember how you learned to drive? Like most people, you probably grew up watching your parents and your older friends drive. By simply watching other drivers, you learned the basic rules of the road and ways to maneuver a car. When you were finally old enough to drive, you began by parking in the driveway as you practiced moving the seat to comfortably reach the pedals, working the blinkers and windshield wipers, and checking the mirrors.

Eventually you were ready to drive on your neighborhood streets. Remember how you carefully put the car in drive, slowly lifted your foot off the brake, and pressed the gas pedal to start moving? Most likely, you pushed the gas pedal too much, then not enough, then too much, hopping along the road like a kangaroo. Signaling while steering into a turn was harder than signaling while parked in the driveway, and sharing the road with other cars was a little scary. Suddenly you realized that while watching people drive had been a great education, driving didn't come as naturally as you'd thought it would. You probably worried you'd never master it.

But as your driving lessons continued, you gradually overcame your early problems and worries. The more you drove, the more a lot of things—like accelerating and braking smoothly, flicking on the blinkers and wipers, and knowing where you needed to be on the road—became automatic. Your confidence grew each day. Within a few months, you could just get in the car and confidently drive with little thought about how it all worked.

Just like driving, breastfeeding is part art and part method. Watching other women breastfeed is vital to understanding how it works, and practicing skills, such as positioning techniques, during pregnancy can be a big help. And while learning how to breastfeed can be more challenging than you imagine, it does get easier with practice.

However, there's one big difference between learning to drive and learning to breastfeed: While nearly everyone has grown up watching other people drive, very few people today have seen breastfeeding firsthand. As you'll learn in Chapter 1, when childbirth moved from the home to the hospital at the beginning of the twentieth century, formula-feeding began to replace breastfeeding as the primary means of infant feeding. In many Western cultures, 80 to 90 percent of babies were formula fed by the 1970s.

Thankfully, concerned health care professionals and parents have brought breastfeeding back to the forefront over the last thirty-five years as the best—and only—way to feed babies. Unfortunately, this fact still remains: Many of today's women are highly motivated to breastfeed, but they're short on confidence because they haven't had a chance to learn breastfeeding skills. If you ask the average pregnant woman how she'll feed her baby after he's born, she might answer, "I'll breastfeed—if I can." If you then ask this mother-to-be, "How were you fed as a baby?" her answer would most likely be, "I was formula-fed." For many women, learning how to breastfeed is like getting behind the wheel without ever having seen someone drive.

Even if you've seen breastfeeding firsthand, you may still find yourself short on confidence at times—especially early on. Chances are, you've seen experienced mothers smoothly breastfeeding rather than new mothers awkwardly working their way through the learning process. If you've watched an experienced mother, she probably lifted her shirt and simply popped the baby on to her breast. The mother sat and chatted with you, occasionally looking down to smile or caress her baby, but not really appearing to concentrate on helping the baby latch or continue sucking. Watching this unfold, you may have secretly said to yourself, "Breastfeeding—I can do that!" because it looked so easy and "natural." Such encounters may motivate you to breastfeed and help you recognize mastery of breastfeeding, but they don't teach you the practical skills you need to reach that goal yourself.

So how do you learn to breastfeed, then? This book will help you. It's a "crash course" to give you the skills and confidence once passed down through the generations. You may imagine you'll use this book only after your baby is born—because many mothers don't pick up breastfeeding guides until they face a problem—but the best time to read and learn all you can about breastfeeding is while your baby is growing beautifully inside you. You'll learn how to practice proper positioning and prepare for that first important feed after your baby is born. You'll also learn how to avoid many common complications and how to quickly overcome the problems you do encounter.

For simplicity, I've written most of the book for women expecting a first and single baby, but if this isn't your first baby or if you're having twins—or more—I'm sure you'll still find it informative. Also, the book frequently mentions a partner, but it'll still be helpful if you're parenting alone. The basics of breastfeeding are the same for most women, but mothers with more than one child and mothers without partners may need extra help—and patience—to make breastfeeding work.

Throughout the book you'll find special tips and insights. The text boxes with the key icon highlight information that's key to having a positive breastfeeding experience and becoming a skillful and loving mother. The "Things to Do" sections include practical suggestions for specific situations. You'll also find many delightful, insightful letters to me in which real moms share their wisdom and experiences.

While this book addresses many common and uncommon breastfeeding issues, I didn't set out to detail every phase of breastfeeding nor every possible problem. This is a simple resource guide meant to give you confidence rather than a comprehensive reference that might overwhelm and frustrate you. If you encounter an issue that's not covered here, contact a breastfeeding counselor at a support group such as La Leche League International or a lactation consultant for support and advice. (When you seek help from a lactation consultant, make sure she has the world-recognized International Board Certified Lactation Consultant [IBCLC] credential.) You'll also find many other helpful resources throughout the book and a Recommended Resources section at the end.

I hope this book gives you the confidence to provide your baby the very best by breastfeeding. If you have problems in the early days, you may be upset and tearful, and you may lose some confidence because you thought breastfeeding would be easy and natural. Keep in mind that the only natural part is making the milk, which your body does automatically. The practical art of breastfeeding takes commitment and practice, and it may very well take you a few days or weeks to master it. This book will sustain you through that time. As the days go by, you'll become more and more confident, and you'll watch your baby thrive on your milk and love.

What You Need to Know about Breastfeeding

How Breasts Work

Breasts are very interesting parts of your body! Understanding how they work, including how they change during pregnancy and after birth, will help you feel positive about breastfeeding. Your breasts go through four main stages to prepare for breastfeeding:

Stage 1: Embryonic and Fetal Changes

By six weeks into your mother's pregnancy, you had "milk lines" of breast tissue from each armpit to your groin. As you continued to develop and grow, your breast tissue and nipples migrated to their current places on your chest. It's possible to have nipples or breast tissue anywhere along the original milk lines. In fact, it's quite common for women to have breast tissue in their armpits that fills up with milk when prolactin hormone levels rise during the first week postpartum. If you have this extra breast tissue, it won't affect how your true breasts make milk. The milk in the extra tissue can't drain out through your true breasts, so it'll take two to four weeks for your blood system to reabsorb the milk. You can reduce the swelling by applying a cold pack and gently rotating your arms to improve lymph and blood flow in that area.

Stage 2: Puberty Changes

At birth, female and male breasts are the same. Hormonal changes at puberty and during your menstrual cycles further developed your female breasts for breastfeeding. During the months before your first period, your body began producing estrogen and progesterone hormones, and you experienced some breast growth. Since then a small amount of breast growth has occurred during each menstrual cycle. This growth continues during each cycle until about age thirty.

Stage 3: Pregnancy Changes

You might have noticed breast changes before you even realized you were pregnant. In the first trimester (the first three months) of pregnancy, nipples and breasts are often very tender. In the second trimester, nipples and areola (the darker skin around the nipple) become larger and more deeply pigmented. Many hormones are involved in the growth of the milk-making sacs and ducts in your breasts. The most important of these are the placental hormones: estrogen, progesterone, and human placental lactogen. Prolactin is also important to breast growth, and from twelve weeks on, it helps you produce a small amount of colostrum (the first milk) in your breasts. However, high levels of progesterone keep your body from making large amounts of milk until your baby is born and you deliver your placenta. At that point, the real milk-making begins.

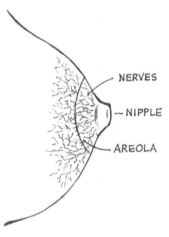

NERVES

— NIPPLE

AREOLA

Breast Size and Lack of Breast Growth

You can't predict the amount of milk you'll make by the size of your breasts. Small and large breasts work the same way: Your breasts will simply make as much milk as your baby (or a breast pump) takes out of them. If your breast size doesn't change during pregnancy, it doesn't mean you'll have problems making milk. Frequent feeding, which your baby will want during the early weeks, will keep high levels of prolactin in the small milk sacs in your breasts, which will ensure you'll make enough milk.

However, if you have very little or no breast growth as well as a thyroid disease (hypothyroidism) or other endocrine gland problem (such as polycystic ovarian syndrome), then it's important to discuss your situation with a lactation consultant or your caregiver. Your caregiver may need to start you on a hormone treatment or increase the amount of the hormones you're taking to assist breast growth during pregnancy and milk production after your baby is born.

Stage 4: Postpartum Changes

Once you deliver the placenta and your blood progesterone level drops, the main breastfeeding hormone, prolactin, will start the milk-making process. Oxytocin is the other exciting hormone your body will release when you begin breastfeeding. Oxytocin is the most wonderful of hormones. It's the hormone of:

- love
- labor
- lactation

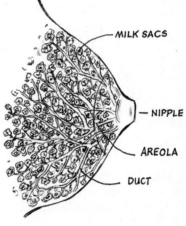

When you're involved in any of these activities, your body releases varying amounts of oxytocin into your bloodstream. During acts of love—such as kissing, lovemaking, and orgasm—oxytocin flows through your body, giving you energy to be very physical as well as bringing wonderful tenderness toward your partner. During natural labor, your body releases huge amounts of oxytocin, causing your uterus to contract and push your baby out. Oxytocin brings you superhuman strength during childbirth as well as incredible feelings of joy and gentleness as soon as your baby is born.

Your baby's early skin-to-skin contact and sucking stimulate the nerves in your breasts and nipples, which tell your body to release more oxytocin. The oxytocin makes the small basket of muscles around your milk sacs contract and push colostrum out of the sacs and down the milk ducts. This is called the milk ejection or letdown reflex. The colostrum then flows out of your breast through nipple pores (the tiny holes at the tips of your nipples) and into your baby's mouth. Because oxytocin also makes you feel tenderness toward your baby, you'll probably find yourself caressing him as he feeds.

When your baby latches on to your breast, he needs to open his mouth wide to take in as much breast as possible, so he'll stimulate the numerous nerves entwined around the blood vessels beneath your areola. This will send a message to your brain for prolactin (the milk-making hormone) and oxytocin (the milk-flow hormone) to come back to your breast via your blood supply. If your baby is premature or can't feed at the breast in the early days or weeks for some other reason, frequent expressing will stimulate these nerves, increase your prolactin level, and build your milk supply until your baby is ready to breastfeed.

As your body gets used to breastfeeding, you'll release oxytocin and your milk will flow as soon as your baby is close to your breast. As the weeks go by, you may even find that your milk will flow when you hear any baby cry or when you talk about your baby, even if he's not with you.

Breast Surgery

Many women have breast surgery for breast lump removal, breast reduction, or breast augmentation. If you've had one of these surgeries, you may still be able to breastfeed successfully, depending on how your caregiver did the procedure.

Lumpectomy

Many women have breast lumps removed. One of the problems is that surgeons like to hide the scar by cutting around the edge of the areola. This may cut some important ducts and nerves, which can affect the production and flow of milk as well as nipple and areola sensitivity. If you've lost sensitivity, you may have less milk in that breast and need to stimulate the supply in your other breast. You can certainly make enough milk in one breast as long as your baby drains it frequently so it can refill. If you have a scar farther out on your breast, then the ducts in that area may have been cut, and you may have a small area in your breast where milk can't flow. The rest of the breast, however, will still produce plenty of milk, and you'll have the other breast to use as well.

Breast Reduction

After breast-reduction surgery, most women have an "anchor scar" created when the surgeon first cut around the areola, next cut down from six o'clock on the areola, and then cut in a half-circle around the breast. The shape of the scar is the same whether the surgeon cuts off the nipple or just repositions it, leaving its blood and nerve supply intact.

If your areola and nipples have been cut off and sewn back on, even though you'll still make milk, it probably won't flow through the ducts and out your nipples to your baby. You'll need to discuss with your caregiver how to stop milk production, and he or she may suggest cold packs for your comfort.

If your nipple was repositioned and you still have good nipple and areola sensitivity, you should be able to produce milk and breastfeed your baby. Sometimes the supply is not quite enough for the baby, so you may need to feed your baby donated milk from a milk bank (see page 11) or formula using a supplementer (see pages 76–78) or bottle.

Having previously had breast-reduction surgery, I had the pleasure of partial breastfeeding, but after nine months Fin has decided it's time for a bottle only! Your confidence in my ability to breastfeed was paramount. After being told by a number of health professionals that I couldn't breastfeed, it was hard to overcome my lingering doubts until finally I got some good, practical advice. Breastfeeding with the supplementer was a wonderful experience and was so beneficial in our development. The bond is so special, and I'm hoping I'll have the same opportunity with our next baby, too.

—Lisa

Breast Augmentation

When doing breast-augmentation surgery, surgeons usually make a cut down the side of the breast and over the ribs and then slide the implant in between the breast and the ribs. This means there's little or no interference with the nerve supply to the breast, so nerve messages for the release of prolactin and oxytocin are easily sent to the brain. Some surgeons cut around the areola to insert the implant, but if you've had this procedure and your nipple and areola are sensitive to touch, you can be reasonably sure breastfeeding won't be affected.

Things to Do

✔ If you've had breast surgery, make an appointment to discuss this with your caregiver. He or she will help you contact your surgeon to determine how the surgery was done.
✔ Discuss the use of a supplementer during this visit.
✔ Contact your local breastfeeding support group. They usually stock supplementers and may be able to connect you with other women who've used them.

Human Milk for Human Babies

There are over four thousand species of mammals. Each species makes milk for its offspring's unique development and feeds its babies at different intervals, depending on their unique needs.

The gray seal wants her pup to gain 3.5 pounds a day and to develop a thick layer of blubber to keep it warm. During her three weeks of lactation she eats nothing and loses over 140 pounds as she breaks down her fat to make milk. She feeds her pup with her fat-rich milk (over 50 percent fat) four or five times a day.

The rabbit wants her bunnies to double their birth weight in a week and develop muscle bulk so they can flee from danger when necessary. She feeds her offspring a high-protein milk (20 percent protein) once a day.

The cow wants her calf to double its birth weight in six weeks and produces a milk with 3.5 percent protein to promote quick muscle growth. She feeds her calf every four to six hours. She also likes to leave her calf hidden in the tall grass, so her milk has casomorphins to drug her calf to sleep while she wanders off to graze.

Humans are the most immature of all mammals at birth, and our health and development require natural human nutrition and constant care. Breastmilk and breastfeeding provide both of these. Human milk is an amazing food specially made for human babies. The human mother wants her baby to gain up to an ounce each day and to double his birth weight in twenty weeks. She makes breastmilk, which contains a high level of lactose that will optimize brain and spinal cord growth. She feeds her baby this high-carbohydrate (7 percent), low-protein (0.8 percent) milk eight to twelve times a day.

Human babies don't need lots of fat to stay warm, as gray seal pups do. Their mothers cuddle and clothe them instead. Although fat makes up half the calories in human breastmilk, the important fat components are the essential fatty acids, which are vital for the growth and development of the brain, the nervous system, the fatty myelin sheath that covers the spinal cord, and the eyes.

Human beings, with the most complex brain of all the mammals, also have the highest amount of lactose, a carbohydrate, in their milk. Cow milk has 35 percent less lactose because calves don't need complex brain growth as human babies do. A human baby breaks lactose into glucose for energy and galactose for the development of the brain and central nervous system. Lactose also helps the baby absorb iron and calcium and promotes the growth of lactobacillus, a good bacteria that stops the growth of harmful bacteria in the baby's intestine.

Human mothers don't need to produce high-protein milk for muscle growth, as the rabbit mother does, because human babies don't start crawling until they're around six months old. Human milk protein is very easily digested because it has a soft curd that breaks down very quickly. This means babies need to feed quite frequently—about eight to twelve times every twenty-four hours during the early weeks. The protein in cow milk has a hard curd, which calves slowly digest. This is why babies who are fed formula modified from cow milk often suffer from constipation—the curd is difficult for humans to digest. (For more on formula, see pages 9–10.)

Breastfeeding provides amazing health benefits not only for babies but also for mothers. Breastfeeding encourages the uterus to contract, which reduces postpartum bleeding. It also lowers a mother's risk of suffering from obesity, osteoporosis, ovarian cancer, and premenopausal breast cancer later in life.

The Importance of Colostrum

The first milk made in your breasts is an amazing fluid called colostrum. Colostrum is the thick, concentrated, clear or yellow-orange fluid your baby will drink during the first couple of days before your breasts fill with mature milk. Every mammal baby needs its own species' colostrum at birth because it carries antibodies for immunity. Colostrum is often milked from horses and pigs and then freeze-dried so it can be given to prize or sick foals and piglets to give them the best start in life. Farmers also say that calves and lambs that don't receive colostrum often suffer from diarrhea and do not develop well.

Unbelievably, some people don't have the same high regard for the importance of human colostrum, even though research has shown that many premature babies would have died or would have had digestive tract infections if they hadn't received their mothers' colostrum.[1] Of all mammals, human babies have the least mature immune system at birth and depend the most on the antibodies in colostrum.

In the first forty-eight hours of life, a human baby doesn't need to drink very much at all—half a teaspoon of colostrum at the first feed and one teaspoon per feed by the end of the second day (see pages 46–47). A very small amount of this thick fluid coats the baby's digestive tract and stops bacteria from crossing into his blood supply and infecting him. Indeed, many texts and research papers show that breastfed babies have much fewer infections compared to formula-fed babies.[2]

Colostrum is important to all babies, but it's vitally important to premature babies. For many years I worked in a hospital where the pediatricians asked all mothers with premature babies to express colostrum for as many days as they could, even if they weren't intending to breastfeed (see pages 63–66).

The Hazards of Formula-Feeding

For most of human history, breastmilk was the only nutrition available for babies. Certainly some women chose not to breastfeed, but the majority of their babies still received breastmilk from wet nurses. When babies received the milk of various animals in past centuries, they usually died.

In the late nineteenth century, scientists began creating infant formula by modifying cow milk. By the time doctors moved childbirth from the home to the hospital in the early twentieth century, formula was more readily available to parents. As doctors favored this new "scientific" approach to infant nutrition and as health care practices led new mothers to quickly abandon breastfeeding (see pages 35–36), more and more women formula-fed their babies. Perhaps you yourself were raised on formula.

Formula companies market their products as being as good as breastmilk, but parents and caregivers should think carefully before giving babies even one bottle of formula as an alternative to breastmilk. Studies have shown that powdered formula is not sterile.[3] There's a risk of contamination with *Enterobacter sakazakii* and salmonella, which could cause infection. Just as there are many health risks associated with cow milk formula, the long-term effects of soy formula are unknown. Soy formula contains phytoestrogens, natural components of plant foods that are similar to mammalian estrogens.

As we learn more about the nutrients in breastmilk, such as essential fatty acids, companies add some of these substances to formula to make it more like breastmilk. But we don't know the long-term effects these additives will have on formula-fed babies because they don't work the same way in formula as they do in breastmilk. For example, breastmilk contains both short-chain polyunsaturated fatty acids (SC-PUFAs) and long-chain polyunsaturated fatty acids (LC-PUFAs). Breastmilk has a range of LC-PUFAs,

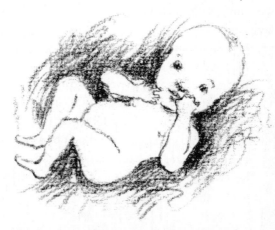

particularly arachidonic acid (AA) and docosahexaenoic acid (DHA), which converts the SC-PUFAs linoleic and linolenic acids for full biological effects. Many types of formula contain only SC-PUFAs, which themselves cannot perform the full range of biological actions. Formula supplemented with AA and DHA additives is available, but medical literature doesn't show whether supplementing formulas with DHA has the intended long-term benefits to formula-fed infants.

As each generation is formula-fed, more health problems arise. Formula-fed babies are more likely to suffer from the following:

- acute diarrhea
- respiratory tract infections
- ear infections
- asthma
- eczema
- rhinitis
- food allergies
- celiac disease
- Crohn's disease
- ulcerative colitis
- IQ deficit of 8.9 points
- juvenile rheumatoid arthritis
- multiple sclerosis
- obesity
- necrotizing enterocolitis
- botulism
- urinary tract infections
- sudden infant death syndrome (SIDS)
- insulin-dependent diabetes mellitus
- childhood lymphomas
- cardiovascular disease later in life

When Mothers Cannot or Do Not Breastfeed

While breastmilk should be the only food for babies in most circumstances, sometimes formula-feeding is encouraged or required for the following health reasons:

- The mother needs major cancer surgery with follow-up therapy.
- The mother has untreated tuberculosis.
- The mother has a high level of hepatitis C, HIV, or HTLV-1 virus.
- The mother needs to take one of the few medications not safe for breastfeeding babies, such as for cancer and certain psychiatric disorders.
- The baby has galactosemia and can't break down galactose, a simple sugar in milk, or the baby has phenylketonuria and can't break down phenylalanine, a component of milk protein. (Most babies get a blood test for these rare conditions in the first forty-eight hours after birth.)

Things to Do

If you need surgery or must take an excluded medication shortly after your baby's birth, ask your caregiver if you can delay the treatment so you can breastfeed or express for the first four or five days of your baby's life. You'll always cherish the joy of having skin-to-skin contact and giving your baby your colostrum and early milk, even if it's only for a short time.

If you have to stop breastfeeding temporarily while you recover from surgery or complete your medication course, then you'll need to express regularly to maintain your milk supply until you're ready to return to breastfeeding. You may be advised to simply "pump and dump" or discard your milk until it's safe to resume breastfeeding.

If you have to permanently stop breastfeeding, the best way to slow your milk supply is to let your breasts get very tight and full and then express them as completely as possible. Prolactin levels decrease whenever breasts are overfull, and this leads to a drop in milk production. Over the next two or three days, keep expressing them as completely as possible whenever they get really tight, increasing the time between expressing until your breasts stop making milk. You may find you'll still have small amounts of milk for some weeks or months.

In most of these situations, caregivers advise mothers not to breastfeed because they'll pass either drugs or viruses to their babies via their milk. The healthiest option for the babies in such cases is to be fed breastmilk from a milk bank. Donor milk banks use the same screening methods as blood banks to ensure that infections are not passed onto the babies who receive the milk. Mothers who donate their milk are also carefully screened for health behaviors such as smoking, use of excluded drugs, and alcohol use. The mothers who donate their milk have over-abundant supplies for their own babies, and the milk bank organizes the collecting, screening, storing, and overnight express shipping of the frozen milk to hospitals or directly to needy mothers' homes. To find out if there's a milk bank in your area, visit http://www.hmbana.org/index.php?mode=locations. When donated milk is not available, babies need formula.

Though some women (or their babies) have serious health issues that prevent them from breastfeeding, many women are discouraged from breastfeeding or never even try it due to a lack of knowledge, support, and assistance. If your mother and grandmother were advised not to breastfeed or didn't receive proper breastfeeding support, they may lament the rules enforced when they were new mothers or not understand why you're being taught different ways of caring for your baby. If you have a sister or friend who had to give up breastfeeding because of a health issue or because she couldn't overcome an early problem, she may feel guilty or defensive about having to formula-feed.

Instead of harboring negative feelings, it's more productive to acknowledge and understand how medical practices worked against breastfeeding for many years—and in some cases, still work against it today. Many women don't reach their breastfeeding goals because their hospitals and clinics lack staff with the necessary expertise to help women overcome breastfeeding difficulties. For example, even with obstacles such as a lack of breast growth due to polycystic ovarian syndrome or the removal of too much breast tissue during breast-reduction surgery, mothers can still give some breastmilk to their babies, but some caregivers aren't able or willing to provide the necessary support and encouragement. The lack of support and knowledge from the medical community seeps into our everyday lives as well. Some women never even attempt to breastfeed because marketing leads them to believe formula is "just as good" as breastmilk. Also, they may have seen breastfeeding portrayed only in a sexual or negative way on TV or in movies, or they may have heard only horror stories about how difficult and painful it can be.

Choosing how to feed your baby is a very personal decision—one all parents must make for themselves. But that decision can be much easier when you have proper knowledge about breastmilk and proper support to reach your breastfeeding goals. Research has shown that women can more easily overcome breastfeeding difficulties and breastfeed for a much longer period when they learn as much as they can about breastfeeding during pregnancy.[4] In the next chapter, you'll learn how to prepare for a successful breastfeeding experience.

Chapter 2

PREPARING FOR BREASTFEEDING

You'll remember that in the Introduction I likened learning to breastfeed to learning how to drive a car. Before you drove for the first time, you probably practiced while parked in your driveway. You turned on blinkers and wipers and found a comfortable driving position. It didn't mean you knew how to drive, but it most likely made learning to drive a little easier.

Likewise, preparing for breastfeeding while you're still pregnant can make the learning process easier once your baby is born. Now's the time to learn about positioning and latching, which may help you avoid some common problems. It's also time to think about your support network, because as you learn to breastfeed and parent, you'll need all the help you can get from friends, family, and professionals. Lastly, it's time to get equipped with items that will make breastfeeding easier (though you may be surprised by how little you really need).

Preparing for breastfeeding during pregnancy is not the same as learning to breastfeed. That's something you can accomplish only with practice after your baby is born. But hopefully the guide to getting started in this chapter can make the learning process easier and more positive for both you and your baby.

Practicing Breastfeeding

Practicing breastfeeding—you might think this is a weird concept! Surely breastfeeding can be done only when you have a baby. You're right: You can't practice the real thing. This type of practice is like an astronaut learning in a simulator. Breastfeeding involves many reflexes and responses, and the more you practice them now, the more relaxed you'll be when you try breastfeeding for real when your baby arrives.

Getting to Know Your Breasts

Most women are modest about their bare breasts. Pregnancy is the time to get to know your breasts better and get used to touching them. When you're breastfeeding, you'll touch your breasts many times every day, and you'll need to be comfortable with that.

The only time some women touch their breasts is in the shower, when they wash and dry them before "putting them away" and forgetting about them for the rest of the day. Many women think about their breasts only during lovemaking and foreplay. Some women get a great deal of pleasure from their breasts during sex and are a bit uncomfortable about using them for a purpose like breastfeeding. Other women associate their breasts with pain because their partners often massage the nipples, thinking this will be pleasurable, when massaging the areola is usually more comfortable and enjoyable. When breast handling has been painful, women tend to have negative feelings about touching their breasts.

Once your nipple and breast tenderness subsides after early pregnancy, you may find it helpful to massage your breasts and areola each day, perhaps in the shower. You can do this gentle massage by cupping your breasts in your hands and gently bringing your thumbs toward your areola and nipples. After this gentle massage, you may want to hand-express a drop or two of colostrum (see pages 20–21), which your breasts start making around the twelfth week of your pregnancy.

You may worry about how breastfeeding will feel. When it's done correctly, it shouldn't hurt at all. As some wise person said: "If sex and breastfeeding weren't pleasurable, we wouldn't have evolved this far." Try this exercise: Put your thumb on one side of your nipple and your forefinger on the other side. Now squeeze. Ouch! Not a nice feeling at all. That's what'll happen if your baby takes only your nipple into her mouth with improper positioning. Now put your thumb on one outside edge of your areola and your forefinger on the opposite edge, push back into your breast towards your ribs, and bring the tips of your thumb and finger together "through" your breast. Was that more comfortable

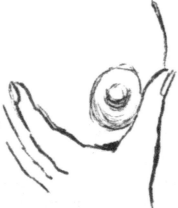

than the ouchy pinch? Breastfeeding shouldn't be painful if your baby takes as much breast into her mouth as possible. This is why it's so important to practice proper positioning as much as you can before the baby arrives.

Positioning and Latching: Step-by-Step Guides

Before you read any further about practicing positioning and latching, it might be helpful to review these terms because they may be new to you. *Positioning* refers to both you and the baby. For you, it simply means finding a comfortable way to sit or lie to feed. For the baby, it means how you'll hold her, and there are many ways to do that. *Latching* is when your baby physically latches her mouth on to your breast to feed. It's something almost all babies instinctively do when placed in a good position.

You can avoid many breastfeeding problems with proper positioning and latching. If you've never closely watched a mother breastfeed, you'll want to practice positioning and latching with a doll. Find a doll you've packed away or borrow one from a friend's child, and try the following step-by-step guides. Your doll obviously won't open its mouth and move like your baby will. But the more you imagine the doll is a real baby, the more you'll learn from these practice sessions and the easier breastfeeding will be when your baby arrives.

For the first important feed after birth, you'll most likely be lying down with your baby on your chest. Your baby will position herself and latch when she's ready (see pages 36–38). At later feeds, you may use the following positions, as shown in the illustrations below: (a) cradle hold, (b) cross cradle hold, (c) "football" hold, or (d) lying down. With cooking, there's more than one recipe for the same dish. With breastfeeding, there's more than one "recipe" for positioning so your baby can easily latch. You may feel like there are too many steps and too much to remember in the following positioning recipes, just as there can be in a cooking recipe. But as I'm sure you know, the more you use a particular recipe, the less you need it.

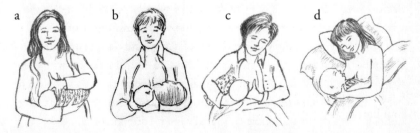

a   b   c   d

Cradle Hold

1. Find a comfortable chair.
2. Decide which breast you'll "feed" from. Lay the doll comfortably on your forearm or in the crook of your arm on the same side you're going to feed from. The doll's head should face your breast.
3. Turn the doll on its side and wrap its body around your body tummy to tummy.
4. Hold the doll very close with its nose pointing at your nipple. You'll need to position the doll so its chin is lifted up and gently pushed into your breast. If this were a real baby, her feeding reflexes would kick in once her chin touched your breast. She would smell your milk and lift her mouth, which would be in exactly the right place to latch.
5. If this were a baby, you'd watch for:
   * her mouth to open wide,
   * her tongue to come forward over her bottom gum, and
   * her bottom lip to turn outward on your breast.

   At this point, bring the doll toward you.
6. Most babies will instinctively latch this way. You can also help by shaping your areola with your first finger on the edge of the areola and your other fingers as far away from the areola as possible. Your fingers will make a V pointing down on your breast. Squeeze your breast so it and your fingers are parallel to the doll's lips.
7. Relax. If you like, support the doll on a pillow after it has "latched." Using a pillow before latching often creates problems with both positioning and latching.

Cross Cradle Hold

If your baby doesn't breastfeed within an hour or so after birth, your caregiver or nurse may want to manually make the baby latch. To do this, he or she would hold the baby's head in one hand and your breast in the other and press your baby's head into your breast. This can very easily lead to breastfeeding difficulties at following feeds (see page 37). In case difficulties occur with the first feed, the following position is a good one to have practiced so you can help your baby latch without creating future problems. Even if you don't have difficulty with the first feed, the cross cradle hold is a good position to know.

1. Find a comfortable chair.
2. Start by practicing "feeding" on your left breast. Lay the doll on its side, facing your left breast and wrapping its body around your body tummy to tummy with your right arm along its back.
3. Support the weight of the doll along your arm with your hand across its shoulders. Put your thumb over one shoulder and your fingers over the other so you don't hold its head. If this were a real baby, she would tilt her head back.
4. Hold the doll very close with its nose pointing at your nipple. You'll need to position the doll so its chin is lifted up and gently pushed into your breast. Again, if this were a real baby, her feeding reflexes and responses would kick in once her chin touched your breast. She would smell your milk and lift her mouth, which would be in exactly the right place to latch.
5. Cup your left hand under your breast. Imagine your breast is a clock with twelve o'clock at the top and six o'clock at the bottom. Place your thumb on the outside edge of your areola at the three o'clock position, and your fingers on the inside edge of your breast (near your breastbone) at the nine o'clock position. Shape your areola, squeezing your breast so it and your fingers are parallel to the doll's lips.
6. Point your nipple to the doll's nose.
7. Rub the underside of your areola on the doll's bottom lip, keeping the nipple above its top lip. As the doll's mouth rubs across your areola, the nipple may become erect and the skin of the areola may crinkle and tighten. Wait until this tightness passes and the nipple and areola are softer before continuing.
8. If this were a baby, you'd watch for:
   - her mouth to open wide,
   - her tongue to come forward over her bottom gum, and
   - her bottom lip to turn down on your breast.

   At this point, bring the doll quickly toward you, with your wrist flat against its shoulder blades.
9. Keep your breast shaped while you imagine the doll taking eight to ten sucks. If it were a real baby, you'd then flip out her top lip with your thumb if it wasn't already turned out. Move your hand away to put it under the doll's body to cradle it.

10. Relax. If you like, support the doll on a pillow after it has "latched." Using a pillow before latching often creates problems with both positioning and latching.

11. Now try on your right breast. Repeat the same steps, only with your left arm along the doll's back and your right hand shaping your breast. This time, your thumb will be at nine o'clock and your fingers at three o'clock, near your breastbone.

> While practicing with the doll, try out different chairs in your home to see which will be the most comfortable while you feed. Different chairs might work better with different positions.

"Football" Hold

Another position to practice while sitting comfortably is the "football" hold. It's called this because you hold the doll much the same way you'd carry a football: The doll is on your arm, tucked at your side, with your hand supporting its head. (Keep in mind that this is like holding an *American* football. For many cultures, "football" is soccer, in which the ball isn't held at all. In those cultures, people often refer to this as the twin hold because most mothers of twins feed with a baby under each arm or as the clutch hold because it's like clutching your handbag under your arm.)

1. Find a comfortable chair. You may want a pillow to support your back and another to support your doll. If you lean forward in this position, you'll get a backache while feeding.

2. Start by practicing "feeding" on your left breast. Place the doll on your left forearm, with its tummy turned against your side, its body draped around your back, and its feet behind you.

3. Cup your breast with your right hand. Imagine your breast is a clock with twelve o'clock at the top and six o'clock at the bottom. Place your thumb on the edge of your areola at the nine o'clock position near your breastbone, and your fingers away from your areola at the three o'clock position. Shape your areola, squeezing your breast so it and your fingers are parellel to the doll's lips.

4. Follow steps 6–10 of the cross cradle hold on pages 17–18. Make sure your wrist is very straight between the doll's shoulder blades. If this were a real baby, that would help her head fall back as you bring her toward you.

5. Now try on your right breast. Repeat the same steps, only with your right arm along the doll's back and your left hand shaping your breast. This time, your thumb will be at nine o'clock and your fingers at three o'clock near your breastbone.

Lying Down

It's important to practice feeding while lying down, as this position allows you to rest while feeding. It comes in especially handy at night. Positioning while lying down might be tricky when the room is dark, you're groggy, and baby is fussy, so it's helpful to practice as much as you can to make those late-night feeds easier.

1. Decide which breast you'll "feed" from. Lie on that side on a bed with your knees bent. Use pillows to support your head and shoulders so you can relax comfortably.
2. Push your bottom back across the bed so you can lay the doll tummy to tummy with you and have its nose clear of your breast. (If you lie with your body straight, you'll find it difficult to tilt the doll's head back for easy latch.) If you're small-breasted, you may find it easiest to position the doll by supporting it with your lower arm. Otherwise, you can simply rest that arm under your pillow, behind your head, or wherever is most comfortable.
3. Place your first and second fingers in a V pointing across your breast, and shape your areola so it and your fingers are parallel to the doll's lips.
4. Follow steps 6–9 of the cross cradle hold on pages 17–18.

> Research has shown that a number of babies have died when they and a parent or other adult have fallen asleep while lying on a couch.[1] Babies can slip between cushions or get trapped against the back of the couch and suffocate. The safest place to lie down to feed is on a bed or on the floor.

As you can see, there are many ways to position yourself and your baby and many ways to hold your breast to help your baby latch. Practice them all, and experiment after your baby arrives until you find what suits you both. Keep in mind that once your baby is born, you may find she won't lie quietly like your doll. Positioning may be difficult when your baby's hands wave around and her head moves back and forth, searching for the right spot to latch. The sooner you notice her feeding cues (see pages 45–46) the better, because positioning and latching can be even more difficult if she's agitated or crying. It's important to calm your baby as much as you can and maybe even wrap her in a receiving blanket with her hands at her sides. (Use a lightweight blanket so you don't have bulky layers of wrap between you.) Once you've learned to respond to her early feeding cues, she'll usually lie quietly and latch easily.

Things to Do

✔ Contact your local breastfeeding support group and plan to attend a meeting with breastfeeding mothers. Watch how the mothers help young babies latch, and see how the older babies just come on and off the breast without help.

✔ Attend a prenatal breastfeeding class and bring your doll to practice positioning with the other women there.

✔ Have your partner watch you practice positioning so you'll have someone to help you remember the steps after your baby is born.

✔ Talk to your lactation consultant or caregiver about positioning and latching. He or she may recommend a helpful video such as *Mother and Baby...Getting It Right* or *Follow Me Mum*.

Expressing by Hand

In addition to practicing positioning and latching, it's also very helpful to practice hand-expressing during your pregnancy. Once your baby is born, if you express a drop or two of colostrum or milk onto your nipple, your baby will smell and lick it, which means she'll have her tongue forward and will be able to latch much more easily. This is how to do it:

1. Place your thumb on the edge of your areola and your fingers on the opposite side of your areola.
2. Push back into your breast.
3. Push your thumb and fingers toward each other through your breast, imagining they're almost going to touch.

4. Relax.
5. Continue the slow squeeze-and-relax steps eight to ten times.

This will be a new sensation, and it may take quite a few practices before you'll feel comfortable. It's usually more comfortable when your breasts are soft and warm during or after your shower. Once you're comfortable, you may find a drop or two of colostrum on your nipple. If you find this expressing practice painful, don't practice again until you've sought advice from your lactation consultant or caregiver. He or she may teach you how to express and may also have the video *Hand Expressing and Cup Feeding* for you to watch.

Learning how to hand-express helps you understand why your baby will need to have her mouth wide open so she can take as much breast as possible into her mouth. If your baby doesn't have enough breast in her mouth, she'll chew your nipple, and she also won't stimulate the nerves around the areola for hormone release. This means you won't make as much milk, your milk won't flow as well, and your baby will want to feed almost constantly in an attempt to get enough food. For more on hand-expressing once your baby is born, see pages 55–58.

Building a Support Network

Practicing positioning and latching techniques before your baby arrives will make it easier to learn the practical art of breastfeeding. Building a good support network during pregnancy will make it easier for breastfeeding to work day by day. A couple generations ago, before suburban sprawl, motherhood was revered by society, and family and close neighbors cared for new mothers for at least forty days after birth. Today things are different. North American families are spread far and wide, and in most communities there are no postpartum customs in place to look after new mothers. It's important to take time now to think about who can help you after your baby is born.

Like many women, you may not feel you'll need support. As part of today's generation of women, you probably balance work, relationships, a household, social commitments, and community involvement, and you pride yourself on your autonomy. If prodded, you may say it'd be *nice* if someone helped you with meals or laundry now and then during the first week, but overall you think motherhood is something you can handle on your own.

Getting help after your baby is born is not just "nice," it's crucial for breastfeeding to work. Breastfeeding takes a great deal of time, patience, and energy to learn. Your baby may feed eight to twelve times in a twenty-four-hour period, leaving you little time for anything else. You'll need someone to take care of household duties so you can rest, as tiredness often leads to breastfeeding problems, particularly mastitis (see pages 102–103). More importantly, you'll need helpful, caring people— whether they're family, friends, or professionals—who support your commitment to breastfeeding and can help you overcome the obstacles you may face.

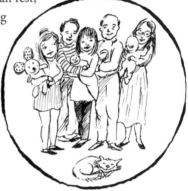

Your Number One Support: Your Partner

Being *partners* means you must see breastfeeding as a partnership. You each play an important role in making it work. Obviously, you must do the physical work of breastfeeding—you provide colostrum and milk for the baby from your breasts. Your partner must support you to make the physical side of breastfeeding easier. Though I certainly don't mean this in an old-fashioned or sexist way, your partner must be your protector and provider. By that I mean your partner needs to protect, support, and provide for you during pregnancy, labor and birth, and breastfeeding.

During pregnancy, your partner must support your commitment to breastfeed and help you prepare so breastfeeding can be easier to learn once the baby arrives. This includes anything from helping you practice positioning to accompanying you to visits with your caregiver or lactation consultant. If your partner is unfamiliar with breastfeeding, as many people are, and is concerned about seeing your breasts in this new way, now's the time to talk through your feelings. If your partner is uncomfortable with the thought of you breastfeeding or can think of your breasts only as sexual objects, it may be difficult to get the full support you need once the baby arrives.

If your partner is unsure about your decision to breastfeed, it often helps to explain the wonderful benefits your baby will receive from your milk. You may also want to visit your caregiver or lactation consultant together to discuss each other's feelings.

Pregnancy is also the time to discuss any concerns your partner may have about how breastfeeding will affect bonding with your baby. Some parents decide not to breastfeed because they feel they can't both bond with their baby if only one can feed. Some breastfeeding mothers express once each day just so their partners can bottle-feed this milk to their babies. If you're considering this as a way to alleviate your partner's worries about bonding, do keep in mind that expressing can be time consuming and bottle-feeding can introduce nipple confusion unless breastfeeding is well established. It's important that you both understand that one of your partner's chief roles is to teach your baby that food isn't the only enjoyment in life. Your baby needs baths, clean diapers, silly play, educational play, as well as hugs, kisses, and snuggles. These are all things your partner can easily provide. Once breastfeeding becomes easier and you return to work or activities outside the home, your partner will have many opportunities to feed your baby your expressed milk.

During labor and birth, your partner will be the person to protect your wishes and needs, which includes your need to have a successful first feed. As you'll learn in the next chapter, you and your baby will need uninterrupted skin-to-skin contact in order to get breastfeeding off to the best start (see pages 36–43). Until the first feed, your partner will have to cuddle you and your baby together rather than hold your baby. This may be difficult, as no doubt your partner will want to hold your baby right away and you'll want your partner to bond with your baby, too. But because breastfeeding is a partnership, you'll both need to do what's best for your new family. That means cuddling as a threesome and leaving your baby with you until the first feed is a success. This also applies to eager grandparents, aunts, uncles, and friends. Your partner can be the one to explain to others why it's important not to pass your baby around for the first twenty-four hours.

After the birth, you'll need a tremendous amount of support, protection, and providing from your partner. This is the time when you'll learn how to breastfeed. You may need protection from visitors, particularly in the early days, when positioning and latching are awkward and you may be uncomfortable breastfeeding in front of guests. Your partner can make things easier for you by politely rustling guests out at feeding time or encouraging them to schedule more convenient visits. As the provider, your partner may also need to be the shopper for a couple of weeks. In the first few weeks, getting yourself ready to go to the store—let alone getting the baby ready, too—can feel as overwhelming as packing and setting off for an international vacation. Let your partner pamper you a little by running errands for you. This will allow you to use whatever free time you have to take a nap, walk, or bath.

Most importantly, your partner needs to provide constant emotional support and encouragement as you learn how to breastfeed. You'll have many ups and downs, many good days and bad days. Some people master breastfeeding in days, some in weeks, and some in months. You may reach a point where it seems easier to give up than to keep going, and that's where your partner can come in to lift your spirits and give you the love and support you need to continue. Likewise, with your partner there to share and celebrate, the little and big victories you'll experience along the way will be even more rewarding.

If You Don't Have a Partner

If you don't have a partner and will be parenting alone, you deserve the same support, protection, and providing as mothers with partners. It just means that building a support network during your pregnancy is a real priority. Try to find as many people as possible to support and help you as a mother. Often a single mother will find one special person—a sister, friend, or her own parent—who can be her "partner" and number one source of support. Parenting on your own is hard work, and learning how to breastfeed can add an extra challenge. Now's the time to reach out to those who can help you. Most people adore babies and will be very keen to help you, especially if they're parents themselves and know what you're going through.

The Breastfeeding Lifeline

Although your partner (or your special support person) can provide a great deal and make breastfeeding easier to master, you'll still need other family and friends to complete your support network. This lifeline exercise was originally developed by Lea Jamieson for special prenatal breastfeeding classes in England.[2] It can help you identify not only your history and familiarity with breastfeeding, but also the areas in which you may—or may not—find support. It's useful if you and your partner each complete a lifeline and talk about the things that emerge.

What to Note on Your Lifeline

Using the lifeline found on page 26, note the following, beginning with your birth up to the present day:

- Note whether you were breastfed or formula-fed. *How you were fed affected how infant feeding was discussed in your family and may affect the type of support you'll receive from your mother. If you don't know whether you were breastfed, this question gives you a good reason to call home. You can talk about the weather and a few other things as well!*
- Note when your siblings (if you have any) were born and how they were fed. *Your position in the family affects your basic parenting knowledge. For example, if you are the eldest of seven, with fifteen years between you and the youngest sibling, then you may have more parenting skills than you'd have if you were the baby of the family or an only child. On the other hand, if you're the youngest in your family, your older siblings can be good sources of support if they already have children.*
- For each of your siblings, friends, and neighbors who are parents, note when they had children and how they fed them. *It can be helpful to know people with babies because you can learn a lot by watching them and going through the same experiences—especially if you're all breastfeeding. If you know people with older children, they can still be supportive because often these parents know what they would do the same and what they would do differently if they could do it all over again.*

You

Birth _____ Today

Your
Partner

Birth _____ Today

A Hypothetical Lifeline

Anna

Birth *I was bottle-fed* *Brother, Michael, was bottle-fed* *Sister, Sarah, was bottle-fed* *Brother, Paul, was bottle-fed* _____ *Friend, Gretchen, breastfed* *Sister, Sarah, breastfed twins* Today

Zac

Birth *I was breastfed* *Sister, Emily, was breastfed* *Sister, Cathy, was breastfed* _____ *Neighbor, Mary, bottle-fed* *Anna's sister, Sarah, breastfed* Today

Anna and Zac have different backgrounds and experiences with breastfeeding, as you can see from their lifelines. When it comes time for Anna to begin breastfeeding, she's likely to be supported by:

- her partner, Zac, who was breastfed and who grew up watching his mother breastfeed his younger sisters;
- Zac's mother, who's an experienced breastfeeder;
- her younger sister, Sarah, who breastfed twins;
- her friend, Gretchen, who breastfeeds her two-year-old daughter and will have a new baby shortly before Anna's baby is due.

Anna is less likely to receive helpful advice from her own mother because she had to wean Anna and did not attempt to breastfeed Anna's younger siblings. Because of her own experience, she may suggest formula-feeding if Anna has even the slightest problem with breastfeeding. Although this can be an emotional and tense situation, Anna needs to keep in mind that her mother most likely didn't breastfeed because she, like many women of her generation, received poor advice from caregivers. She's probably not against breastfeeding—she just has a need and a desire to pass what she knows about feeding and parenting on to her daughter. Realizing this during the pregnancy will allow Anna time to talk enthusiastically to her mother about the fascinating things we now know about breastfeeding and how caregivers are now more trained to help breastfeeding mothers. When the new grandchild arrives, hopefully Grandma will be happy about Anna's decision to breastfeed and eager to support in any way.

Anna and Zac will sit down with each of their support people before their baby arrives to make arrangements for help. Perhaps they'll invite Zac's mother to stay with them for the first week after the baby is born. Perhaps Sarah will stop over in the early evenings with warm meals to help Anna before Zac gets home from work. Perhaps Gretchen will visit in the afternoons so Anna can watch and learn from another breastfeeding mother. Looking at their lifelines, Anna and Zac also remember that Mary, their neighbor, has a nine-month-old. Mary is formula-feeding, so she may not be able to help Anna with breastfeeding issues, but she seems very excited to have a new baby in the neighborhood. Perhaps she can walk over and watch the baby on days when Anna needs a nap. The important thing is that they'll make these plans in advance. Many new parents don't plan for support—and then find themselves on their own, overwhelmed, and unsure of whom to call.

Things to Do

If your mother or partner's mother didn't breastfeed, contact your local breastfeeding support group for helpful booklets about breastfeeding written especially for Grandma. You can give it to her during one of your talks, or you can leave it out on the kitchen counter where she can find it and browse through it.

Beyond Family and Friends

No matter how close-knit your family may be, pregnancy is a time to rekindle and deepen family attachments. Both your and your partner's families will be excited about your coming baby, and their assistance and knowledge may be very valuable. Families are often the foundations of new parents' support networks. Another major source of support is friends, especially when families are scattered. Many new parents seek help from their "family of friends," who often have children around the same age.

If you're approaching parenthood without a network of reliable family and friends, pregnancy is the time to make new contacts and look for other sources of support. Even if you do have family and friends available, it's good to look beyond that network because you can never have too much help.

Other New Parents

If you'd like to meet other expectant or new parents, prenatal classes, baby health care centers, breastfeeding support groups, and playgroups are good places to look. Visit them now, while you're still pregnant, to learn all you can before your baby arrives and also to establish relationships with people who can help with the first weeks of parenthood. Other groups which may have supportive members include:

- craft groups
- cooking classes for expectant fathers
- religious groups
- sporting groups
- adult education classes
- pregnancy yoga or water aerobics classes

Sometimes family and friends give breastfeeding and parenting advice that's meant to be helpful but only adds stress. Some people find it much easier to open up to and seek help from new acquaintances. Regardless of your relationships with friends and family, you may find, as many expectant and new mothers do, that the easiest way to learn about breastfeeding and parenthood is to watch and listen to people who are doing it the same time as you. Friendships often develop from groups like those listed above, and they may continue through the childrearing years.

Lactation Consultants and Other Professional Support

One of the most important members of your support network is your health care professional. Your doctor or midwife or your baby's pediatrician can usually help with some breastfeeding issues, but you may find that a lactation consultant provides the best help and support.

La Leche League International (LLLI), the pioneer breastfeeding self-help group established in the United States in 1956, has led the way in supporting and educating breastfeeding mothers. LLLI has always emphasized mother-to-mother assistance, but it also recognized a need for breastfeeding specialists among health care professionals. LLLI's vision led to the formation of the International Board of Lactation Consultant Examiners (IBLCE), who developed and now oversee the examination for the International Board Certified Lactation Consultant (IBCLC) credential. You can find an IBCLC in your area by visiting the International Lactation Consultant Association (ILCA) website at http://gotwww.net/ilca/.

The rise of the lactation consultant profession over the past twenty years has helped improve how breastfeeding is taught in hospitals, universities, and nursing schools. You can connect with an IBCLC at a hospital, clinic, private practice office, or a home consultation. A few doctors have this special credential as well. An IBCLC can help you overcome any breast-feeding obstacles you discover during pregnancy or any difficulties you face after your baby is born. If you work with an IBCLC, you'll receive well-researched, supportive, and helpful care.

In contrast, many other health professionals aren't as knowledgeable about breastfeeding, and some are actually opposed to it. For many years, infant-nutrition lectures falsely taught medical and nursing students that there was little difference between breastmilk and formula and that formula was a scientific way to "humanize" cow milk. This antibreastfeeding education continues today as formula companies fund health care providers for their continuing education at lavish seminars, conferences, and on-site workshops. Also, formula companies often fund infant-nutrition research, which can affect the researchers' conclusions. Many medical journals receive support from formula companies, and thus advertise their products. In many health care offices, consumers see calendars, pens, and notepads advertising formula, and many people assume the staff supports these products.

In 1981, 118 countries signed the *International Code of Marketing of Breastmilk Substitutes*, recommending that gifts of formula be prohibited in hospitals, but the United States was the only nonsignatory country. In 2005, Massachusetts became the first state in the U.S. to legislate against this practice. This means many North American hospitals still allow companies to give free formula to new mothers leaving the hospital. Some hospitals even allow formula companies to obtain patients' names and addresses—often through photographing babies in the hospital—so they can deliver packs of formula to parents the first week after discharge. Needless to say, this pack can seem quite tempting if it arrives on a day when a mother is tired and discouraged by learning to breastfeed.

If your caregiver doesn't seem to have much infant-nutrition education or seems to have had a negative personal experience with breastfeeding, he or she may not be the best caregiver for you. A negative personal experience can be quite destructive. If the professional is a woman with unresolved breastfeeding difficulties, this may affect her beliefs about breastmilk and her confidence in teaching breastfeeding. If it's a man who's watched his partner struggle with breastfeeding or who felt he did not get enough contact with his baby because his partner was happily breastfeeding, then he may be less supportive in your wish to breastfeed.

Research shows that you need a caregiver—whether a doctor, midwife, or lactation consultant—who uses research-based care and who supports your commitment to breastfeed.[3] If your caregiver seems opposed to or unsure about breastfeeding in any way, you may need to consider finding a new caregiver.

Getting Equipped for Breastfeeding

During pregnancy, many women think "preparing for the baby" simply means buying baby gear. They rush to stores and fill their shower registries with gadgets and gizmos they think will make life with a new baby easier. Actually, baby merchandising is a retailer's license to print money. Advertisements encourage new parents to believe there are many "must have" items. But if you talk to friends who have children, they'll probably say you need to buy very little before your baby is born. It's much better to buy or borrow things as your baby needs them. Your baby will have only a few real needs, especially since you're breastfeeding:

- *Love*: This is naturally supplied—at no expense!
- *Warmth*: Your baby will receive the best warmth from other humans, particularly from your warm, soft breasts as you breastfeed, but she will need some clothes! This doesn't mean you need to buy a lot, because babies grow quickly. Don't underestimate how many clothes you'll receive from relatives and friends. Bibs aren't always necessary for breastfed babies. Even if your baby spits up after a feed, it won't be the sour smell of formula but a sweet smell, so you won't need to change her clothes so often.
- *Food*: Breastmilk is always ready and warm, and it comes in soft, portable, reusable containers. When your baby approaches six months or so, she'll show interest in adding chewable food to her breastmilk diet (see pages 125–126). But until then, all she needs is your milk.
- *Hygiene*: The smell of a breastfed baby is delightful. She doesn't need to be slathered in lotion, nor does she need to be sprinkled with powder. The smell of a formula-fed baby is quite different, which is why parents began using scented powders and lotions. Clean diapers at each feed and an occasional bath are all she'll need.
- *Shelter*: You need to provide a roof over your baby's head, but you may not need to spend much on your baby's bed and bedding—especially in the beginning. You may find it easier and more comforting to bring your baby into your bed or bedroom, particularly while you're establishing breastfeeding. For more on cosleeping and bed-sharing, see pages 79–80.

Getting Equipped: What You Need

Many women wonder if they need to buy special bras for breastfeeding. In the past, women were led to believe their breasts would become droopy if they didn't wear bras day and night from early pregnancy to weaning. However, we now know that wearing bras twenty-four hours a day doesn't lessen the change in breast shape that naturally comes with pregnancy. If you're happy and comfortable without a bra and you don't run into the problem of constantly leaking milk after your baby is born, there's no reason to buy bras. If you need or wish to wear a bra, buy those that make you feel beautiful, supported, and comfortable. There are many designs, and the best of these allow you to completely open the cup for easy access to your breast. Any tightness around your breast while you're feeding may stop your breast from properly draining. If you like to wear a sports bra, you'll need to be careful when you pull it up over your breast because that tightness could also prevent good breast drainage and lead to mastitis.

If feeding in public concerns you, you may want to buy dresses and tops designed with hidden openings so you can breastfeed discreetly. Otherwise, it's not difficult to breastfeed in your usual clothes once you're relaxed about feeding. You can feed discreetly if you lift your top and then drape your clothes around your breast as soon as your baby latches. (See pages 117–118 for more on feeding in public.)

At some point, you'll probably need to express or pump milk to leave for your baby when you're away from her. Some women prefer hand-expressing because it's easy and cheap for occasional needs. All you'll need is clean hands and a clean bottle or storage bag for the milk. Other women prefer to use pumps, particularly if they express frequently, such as when they return to work or activities outside the home. You can choose from manual, battery-powered, or electric pumps, which vary in price and effectiveness. Watch the classifieds in your newspaper to save money on secondhand battery or electric pumps, though it's always wise to buy breast pump attachments or manual pumps new. (See pages 57–58 for details about expressing milk.)

If you're registering for a baby shower, you might want to include on your registry breastfeeding items such as a pump and storage bags, nursing bras and clothes, a footstool, nursing pillows, and breast pads. Don't worry about including bottles, nipples, or pacifiers. Until breastfeeding is well established, these items can introduce nipple confusion and act as "dummies" that affect your milk supply. If you receive them as gifts, you may feel defensive, thinking the gift-giver presumes you won't be able to mange breastfeeding. More likely, it's just a matter of the gift-giver not understanding how breastfeeding works.

The Keys to Successful Breastfeeding

There's a lot to practice and consider as you await the arrival of your baby and the beginning of your breastfeeding experience. Perhaps the best way to have a long and positive breastfeeding experience is to keep a good grip on the following keys to success:

- You really want to breastfeed your baby.
- You have at least one breast. (Many women with only one breast, including mothers of twins, have breastfed their babies.)
- You're committed to overcoming any problems because you know your milk gives your child the best odds of good health.
- Your partner supports and encourages you, and you and your partner are able to be patient and flexible.
- You have supportive family and friends who have breastfed positively, understand how breastfeeding works, and/or support your commitment to breastfeed.
- You are cared for by health professionals who are well-qualified, good teachers, and supportive.

Before you know it, you'll give birth to your baby, and your breastfeeding lessons will begin in earnest the moment she's placed on your chest. Take the time to make sure you're as prepared for that moment as you can possibly be. The moment you meet your baby and begin this beautiful relationship is quite important, as you'll learn in the next chapter.

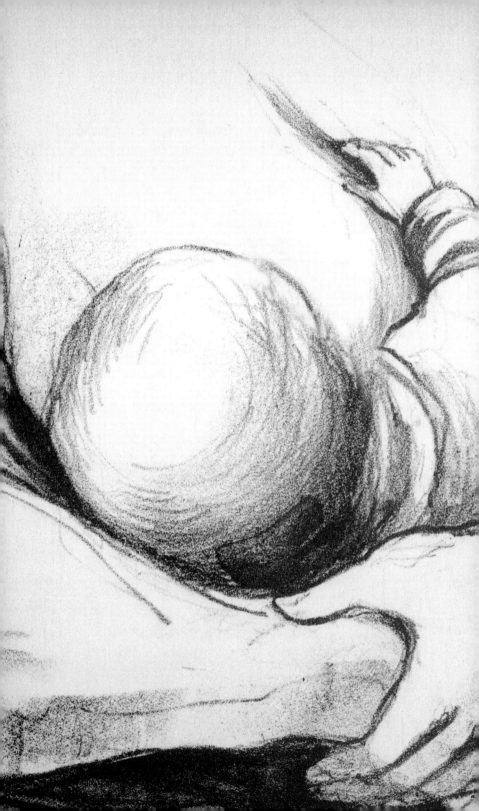

Chapter 3

GETTING OFF TO A GOOD START

Then and Now

I n your great-great-grandmother's day, women gave birth at home and
began breastfeeding immediately, tapping into the knowledge and skill
passed down from woman to woman for generations. Children's doctors
of the day wrote that babies needed to feed twelve times a day for the first
three months and gave little other advice, because mothers knew more about
infant feeding than they did. Then at the beginning of the twentieth century,
medical doctors moved childbirth from homes to hospitals and made new
rules controlling breastfeeding. Many hospital practices throughout the
twentieth century stripped mothers of their confidence, disconnected them
from the wisdom of other mothers, and led them to abandon breastfeeding
within days or weeks.

Babies and mothers were separated during their hospital stays, which
often lasted weeks. Babies would cry in the nursery, waiting to be fed, and
mothers would cry in their beds. Doctors put babies on feeding schedules
with only five feeds a day, which wasn't enough food for hungry babies and
wasn't enough stimulation for mothers' breasts to make sufficient milk over
the long term. Even with little stimulation, mothers' breasts filled with
mature milk, but the reduced feeding schedule left the mothers' breasts full and
painful and led to sore nipples because the babies couldn't latch properly.
Favoring more "scientific" means of infant nutrition, doctors subjected the
babies to test-weighing to determine if they had drunk the "right" amount,
and they made mothers offer complementary bottles of formula after each
feed. It's easy to imagine how these hospital practices affected new mothers'
confidence in their ability to parent and breastfeed. Most women in your
grandmother's and mother's generations quickly gave up breastfeeding after
bringing their babies home.

The good news is: Many of these harmful hospital practices have changed over the past thirty-five years. This change first came about with the insistence of parents armed with up-to-date knowledge from books and breastfeeding support groups, particularly La Leche League International (LLLI). These parents were also supported by well-informed midwives and nurses who started obtaining the International Board Certified Lactation Consultant (IBCLC) certification in the mid-1980s. Once these lactation consultants began working in hospitals, they fostered major changes in hospital policies, such as keeping mothers and babies together for skin-to-skin contact until the first feed, rooming-in, no formula-feeding unless mothers consented, and no gifts of formula as mothers left the hospital. Because of these reforms, you should have a much more positive and encouraging experience in the hospital than your mother and grandmother had, but you may still encounter some problematic hospital practices. (That is, *if* you give birth in a hospital. More often than not, giving birth at home or in a birth center leads to less intervention in birth and early parenting.) You still need to consult with your caregiver during pregnancy in order to make your wishes known ahead of time. This chapter can help you make the most of your hospital stay and get breastfeeding off to a good start.

The First Feed

The first feed is the most important key to successfully starting breastfeeding. When your baby learns how to latch on to your breast for the first time, he "programs" his "computer" to do the same thing whenever the breast is offered. Studies have shown that the earlier his computer is programmed, the fewer difficulties you'll have with breastfeeding. If all goes well, the first feed may happen within a half hour—or it may take two to three hours before your baby is ready. It's vitally important to have uninterrupted body contact with your baby after birth. During this time, your baby's feeding reflexes and responses are heightened, and if left on your chest, he'll find your breast, latch, and feed beautifully on his own.

If you're lying down for the first feed, then your baby will move himself around and find a comfortable position on his own. You don't need to use any special positioning techniques. A particularly informative video, *Delivery Self Attachment* by Lennart Righard and Margaret Alade, shows hour-old babies using their elbows to crawl up their mothers' bodies to their nipples, much as seals use their flippers to move up the beach.

Babies are born with a very active reflex, called the rooting reflex, which they use to search for their mothers' nipples. Before feeding, your baby holds his tongue up against the roof of his mouth. When his chin touches your breast, his feeding reflexes will kick in. He'll move his head backward and forward, searching with his mouth until he finds your areola. As he does this, he'll drop his tongue from the roof of his mouth, open his mouth wide, and gradually extend his tongue over his bottom lip to lick your breast and nipple. Licking is the vitally important first step in learning how to breastfeed. You need to be patient and not hurry him. The more he searches with his tongue, the more of your breast he'll take into his mouth. You may be able to help him a little by bunching up your areola between your first and second finger, making sure your fingers are parallel to his lips and not too close to your nipple.

Some mothers find that the cross cradle hold, which you practiced in the last chapter (see pages 16–18), helps their babies latch more easily. If you try this position for the first feed, just be careful not to put your hand on your baby's head or let your caregiver or nurse push your baby's head to your breast, even if he or she feels you and your baby need assistance. This can very easily lead to breastfeeding difficulties at following feeds. Pushing the baby's head doesn't give him time to learn the important steps of opening his mouth wide, bringing his tongue forward, and licking your breast. It also means his chin won't touch your breast and stimulate his feeding reflexes. Also, your baby may be frightened when someone pushes his head into your breast, and he may later refuse to feed. If you want to help your baby latch with the cross cradle hold, be sure that you support him by the shoulders, as directed.

The first feed not only programs your baby's computer and makes the following feeds easier for him, but it also programs your own computer by telling your body breastfeeding is beginning. Early skin-to-skin contact and sucking stimulates your breasts and nipples, which leads to the release of more oxytocin in your body. This ensures that the letdown (milk ejection) reflex occurs so colostrum flows. Oxytocin release also helps your placenta separate from your uterus if it hasn't already done so, and helps the uterus contract to slow your blood loss. Uterine contractions will continue at every feed until you wean, and they are very important for a healthy uterus. Mothers who don't breastfeed lose blood for a longer time postpartum, making them more susceptible to anemia. If this is your first baby, you may not even notice these contractions at the first feed, but you'll need to change your sanitary pad. You may need a warm pack on your belly to reduce the discomfort in the first few days after your baby is born.

Now's the time, while you're still pregnant, to make plans so the first feed is a memorable experience for you both. An important step is to understand how your baby's senses play a role in his first feed.

Your Baby's Senses and the First Feed

Your baby will use all his senses—sight, smell, taste, touch, and hearing—to position himself, latch, suck, and continue feeding shortly after birth.

Sight

During the first hours, your baby will have a quiet alert phase and will prefer to look at round objects.[1] His eyes will be wide open. When your baby is lying on your chest or in the crook of your arm, he can see your face perfectly. Your baby needs to be less than eight inches away from your face to see you well. If you watch him, you'll see his eyes moving around, taking in every feature of his mother's beautiful face. When you cuddle as a threesome, your baby will also scan your partner's lovely face. Your baby will also notice your round areola. Researchers have suggested that the areolas and nipples darken during pregnancy to help babies see them more easily.[2]

Smell

During your pregnancy, your baby floats around in amniotic fluid. When he's born, he'll be covered in this fluid, which mothers find has an attractive smell and has been shown to assist in bonding.[3] Most of the fluid will be dried off so he doesn't get cold, but the scent will remain. As he lies on your chest, he'll move his hands across your chest and breasts, leaving the amniotic smell there to help him find his way to the breast at later feeds.

Your Montgomery's follicles, those pimple-like bumps on your areola, produce a substance called sebum that not only lubricates your nipples and areola but also has an enticing smell. Your baby will learn this smell as well as your body smell and the smell of your colostrum so he can recognize you. Other newborn animals learn about their mother through a pheromone or scented chemical the mother exudes. Researchers are studying whether human mothers release pheromones as their oxytocin rises when babies' tiny fists and fingers massage their breasts.[4] Studies show that babies prefer their mothers' unwashed breasts to those that have been washed.[5] So if you shower or bathe after the first hour or two, don't wash your breasts, and use perfume sparingly. Research has shown that babies have such a finely tuned sense of smell that they don't feed well if their mothers change their perfume, deodorant, or even laundry detergent.

Because smell is such an important part of breastfeeding after birth, it's important to avoid confusing your baby with too many scents. It's customary for new mothers to hand their babies around to grandparents or other family members and friends in the early hours after the birth. For the first twenty-four hours, only you and your partner should handle the baby (and your partner should wait until after the first feed). If other people cuddle your baby during this crucial early time, they'll leave other smells—food, perfume, after-shave, or cigarette smoke—on his clothes. This will confuse your baby, delay his recognition of you, and interfere with his ability to breastfeed.

Taste

We know that babies like sweet tastes. Drops of colostrum encourage them to lick and become eager to feed. If you haven't learned how to hand-express during your pregnancy (see pages 20–21), ask your caregiver to show you how to express a drop or two of colostrum to give your baby a taste of what your breasts have to offer. As your baby licks the colostrum from your areola and nipple, he learns not only how your milk tastes but also that interesting things happen when he stretches his tongue out.

At about ten weeks into your pregnancy, your baby began to drink the amniotic fluid around him. By forty weeks, he'll have drunk up to a pint each day. This fluid tastes like what you've been eating, which helps him learn what your milk will taste like. This means you don't need to change your diet once you start breastfeeding. An old wives' tales says you can't eat anything with herbs and spices if you breastfeed—and it makes you wonder how babies in Mexico, India, and Thailand cope! If your pregnancy diet includes garlic and chili, then these are tastes your baby will recognize and like in your milk.[6] Babies will drink other mothers' milk, such as donated milk from a milk bank, but they prefer their own mothers' milk because it tastes familiar.

Hearing

Your baby needs calm, quiet time after birth so he can listen to your voice and your body sounds. As your baby lies on your chest, he'll hear the soothing rhythmic heartbeats he listened to for all those months inside you. He'll also hear encouraging words from you. Researchers used to believe the watery sounds of the uterus muffled voices during pregnancy, but new studies have shown that your baby actually hears voices clearly. [7] He'll become very relaxed when you talk to him—he'll lower his breathing rate, and if he's sucking, he'll slow down to listen. If you have a premature baby who must stay in the hospital, it's important to make a tape of you talking so your baby can listen to it when you're not there. This is especially important if the nurses in the nursery do not speak the same language as you, because your baby won't recognize the unfamiliar sounds of their speech.

Touch

Touch is perhaps the most important sense involved in a successful first feed. This is why you and your baby need unrestricted skin-to-skin contact from the moment after birth. Research has shown that when babies have skin-to-skin contact with their mothers, they all follow the same pattern of hand movements to find and stimulate their mothers' breasts.[8] As your baby lies on your chest, he'll gently rub your nipple and areola with his fingers or fists, concentrating on one breast. You might find he'll put his fingers in his mouth to wet them with saliva before he rubs your nipple. As he continues to rub your nipple and areola, your body will release extra oxytocin, helping colostrum flow for him to drink when he's ready.

I see women who had breastfeeding problems with their first babies come into the hospital planning to breastfeed their second babies for only a couple feeds and then "see what happens." They bring formula and bottles, expecting difficulty. It's wonderful to see many of them confidently and happily breastfeeding a few days later. For many of these mothers, having unrestricted skin-to-skin contact after birth plays a major part in ensuring problem-free breastfeeding.

Skin-to-skin contact is also important because the softness and the warmth of your body will be very soothing and relaxing for your baby. While lying on your chest, his heart and breathing rates will drop and become regular.[9] Your body temperature will rise to warm him if he gets a little cold; conversely, if he gets too warm, your body temperature can drop to cool him back to normal temperature. (Still, it's very important that you cover his body with a warm blanket because newborns can become very sick if they get cold.)

Research has shown that if caregivers separate babies from mothers for weighing, dressing, and testing, they take longer to learn how to suck. For this reason, it's very important to have your caregiver do as many observations and treatments as possible, such as the Apgar test and vitamin K injection, while you're skin-to-skin. It's also important not to weigh your baby until after the first breastfeed—even if that's hours after he's born. When it's safe to weigh him, ask the caregiver to lay him on his tummy on a warm cloth. Babies are often weighed bare and on their backs, which makes them cold, frightens them, and brings on their Moro (startle) reflex and stress hormones. Stress hormones reduce babies' ability to use their brown fat for warmth and energy (see page 44), and that lowers their blood sugar. This may lead your baby's caregiver to order formula to raise his blood sugar.

Unrestricted skin-to-skin contact also means relatives and friends need to wait at least until after the first feed—ideally, after the first twenty-four hours—to hold your baby. After the first feed, you'll probably want your partner to have some skin-to-skin contact with your baby. Babies often go into a deep sleep after the first feed, and this is a perfect time for you to shower and dress or perhaps curl up and have a well-earned sleep of your own. Your partner will love this time, and you'll love to see the joy on your partner's face while snuggling with your beautiful child.

> As Ben's dad, I loved the time I spent cuddling with him, and he always looked and felt so warm and comfortable there on my chest. Every father should be urged to do it when his partner is showering, sleeping, or needing time for other things. I don't know if he knew who I was, but for me, holding my son against me was and is a beautiful time for us.
>
> —John

How to Plan for a Successful First Feed

Creating the right conditions for a successful first feed will make breastfeeding much easier, but it's not something that happens on its own in most hospitals. First you'll need to find out what normally happens at your birth site in the hours after a baby is born and also talk to your caregiver about his or her own experiences. (Again, if you give birth at home or in a birth center, you won't run across the same policies as you'll find in a hospital.) If the hospital and your caregiver seem unwilling to support your needs for the first feed, then recruit a midwife or lactation consultant who can obtain the research papers listed in the Recommended Resources on the importance of skin-to-skin contact. You can either have your caregiver read these papers or have the lactation consultant circulate them at the hospital for other staff to learn from. Also ask them if you can watch the video *Mother and Baby...The First Week* together.

Some parents like to write a plan for their caregiver and hospital staff similar to the one below.

Our Plan for the First Hours

- We ask that our baby be dried and covered with our blanket and hospital bedding while having skin-to-skin contact on Mom's chest.
- We ask that the staff do as many observations and treatments as possible for our baby while he's skin-to-skin with Mom.

- We ask that the staff not weigh our baby until after his first breastfeed, even if that is hours after the birth.
- We ask that the staff weigh our baby lying on his tummy on a warm cloth.
- We ask that Dad can cuddle with the baby and Mom on the bed.
- We ask that Dad can cuddle our baby skin-to-skin if Mom is showering, using the bathroom, or is otherwise unavailable.
- We prefer that other relatives and friends do not cuddle our baby in the first twenty-four hours.

I breastfed our twins from the start, although it didn't go quite how I'd hoped in the labor ward—the nurse attached the twins for me (both at once with the twin hold), but Erin really wasn't ready to feed. While I was cleaning up, they put the babies in their bassinet in my room. My husband made a video of Erin at this time, and she was mouthing about, all bundled up. I didn't see this until some weeks after her birth and felt quite sad about it. That's when she should have been with me! But I can't dwell on that. We've certainly made up for it, and I can't beat myself up for things I can't change, can I? Still, I feel sad when I watch the video!

—Rachael

The Next Twenty-Four Hours

You'll rejoice as you and your baby lie in unrestricted skin-to-skin contact and as he makes some effort to have his first feed. All babies are different. Some will just lie at the breast comforted by your warmth and sounds, others will latch for only a few minutes and fall asleep, and many will feed on and off for an hour or so and then go into a deep sleep for many hours. The first feed is just the beginning! The next feed may be an hour later, he may feed every two to three hours for the rest of the day, or he may have a long sleep and not want to feed again for six to eight hours. There's no reason he shouldn't have this long break between the first and second feed, as long as he's not premature; you didn't have problems during your labor and his birth; and his temperature, heart, and breathing rates are normal. After this long break, he'll probably feed every couple of hours, and the hospital staff will encourage you to feed at least every four hours both in the hospital and at home.

The Hibernation Period

The most important organ in your baby's body is his brain, and it requires a constant flow of oxygen-rich blood in the first forty-eight hours after birth. To help this happen, your baby's digestive system needs to be in a hibernation-like state. This means:

- You'll still need lots of skin-to-skin contact with your baby.
- Your baby will have a special fat, called brown fat (brown adipose tissue), around his neck and shoulders as well as around his liver and kidneys. He'll slowly break this down for heat and energy.
- His tummy will still contain some of the high-protein amniotic fluid he's been drinking since about ten weeks into your pregnancy.
- He'll pass only a small amount of urine, as his kidneys do not excrete water at this time.
- You'll make very small amounts of "salty" colostrum, which will stop him from sweating too much, pass on immunity to him, and make him sleepy to conserve his energy.
- The small amounts of colostrum will help your baby learn how to coordinate his sucking, swallowing, and breathing, so he'll be ready for the larger amounts of milk that will start in the next day or two.

At each feed, your baby needs to suck for long periods from one or both of your breasts to help drain the thick colostrum. You can do *either* of the following:

- You can let him suck on the first breast until he's satisfied and detaches himself, and then you can offer the other breast at the next feed.
- If he sucks without swallowing for long periods on the first breast, you can detach him after twenty to thirty minutes, offer the other breast, and then start the next feed with the breast on which he finished.

Once your baby has been through the important hibernation period of the first forty-eight hours, your colostrum will begin changing to milk.

Learning Feeding Cues

This is an important time to learn about your new baby and "condition" your breasts to the feeding pattern: Your baby gives you feeding cues, you pick him up, you sit or lie down to feed, and your milk flows. Your letdown reflex will occur even before feeds once your body becomes used to the feeding pattern. In the days when babies and mothers were separated at hospitals, mothers could not experience the feeding pattern. Instead, nurses brought their crying, frantically hungry babies in from the nursery. This meant it took quite a while for their milk to flow—if it flowed at all. Now that mothers and babies room-in at the hospital, you'll learn your baby's feeding cues right away, your letdown reflex will work quickly, and your milk will flow as soon as your baby requires it. (And if you're at home or in a birth center, you'll most certainly have constant contact with your baby so you can learn this important pattern.)

Here are the cues to look for, beginning with the early, calm cues and continuing to the later, stressed cues. As you can imagine, the earlier you respond to your hungry baby, the better.

Early Cues

One of the first things you'll learn about your baby is that he's very clever—he can tell you he's hungry without making a sound:

- He'll start to wriggle, moving his arms and legs around.
- He'll move his head from side to side, searching for you and your breast, even if he's not on your chest.
- He'll put his fingers in his mouth as he did soon after birth.

You'll need to have your baby close in order to see and respond to these early cues so he doesn't move into despair. Pick up your baby quickly at this point, and don't change his diaper or clothes until he's had part of his feed to keep him calm. The more stressed he becomes, the harder feeding will be.

Stressed Cues

If you haven't been close enough to see the early cues, your baby will move on to more stressed cues:

- He'll become fussy and start to make squeaky noises.
- His wriggling will increase as he becomes restless, and he'll let out some short cries.
- Finally, he'll start to cry and scream until he becomes red in the face. He won't want to be positioned, and he may even push you away and refuse to latch.

If your baby frets and cries frequently, and it doesn't seem linked to hunger, it might mean he hasn't latched well during his first couple of feeds. This frustration won't be because he hasn't had enough to drink but because his lips haven't turned outward against your breast as he feeds. The insides of our lips have many sensory nerves that send messages to our brain. As adults, these nerves react to a passionate kiss by making us light-headed. This is due to oxytocin being released into the brain, which lowers blood pressure and calms us. The same should happen for your baby when your breast massages the inside of his lips. Oxytocin and another calming hormone called cholecystokinin will be released, and he'll feel calm, full, and sleepy. Without these hormones, your baby may fret and constantly search for the breast, which may make you think he's hungry.

Feeding on Demand

As you watch your baby for feeding cues throughout the first two days, you may wonder whether you're feeding him too often or not enough. There are no schedules to breastfeeding. Most breastfed babies feed eight to twelve times each twenty-four hours and often not at the same times or at regular intervals. Here's a guide to what your baby takes in and puts out:

First Twenty-four Hours

- Half a teaspoon of colostrum each feed
- Green-black stool
- One wet diaper

Second Twenty-four Hours

- One teaspoon of colostrum each feed
- Soft green-brown stool
- Two wet diapers

Your caregiver should encourage you to let your baby's needs rather than a mandatory schedule regulate feeds. This wasn't true for the women of your mother's and grandmother's generations. At the beginning of the twentieth century, one eminent child-nutrition expert—who happened to be a dairy farmer—suggested that just as cow milk has lower fat when calves feed too often, human breastmilk must have lower fat when babies feed too often. So by the 1920s, mothers in hospitals were taught to feed their babies only every four hours and to have an eight-hour gap at night. Some children's health booklets of the time showed how babies should fill in their day (see graph to the right).

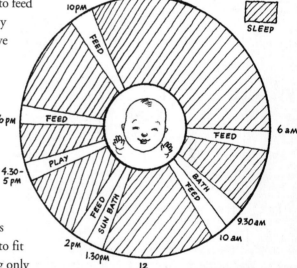

As you can imagine, new mothers felt that they needed to fit this pattern of feeding only five times in twenty-four hours in order to have nice, smiley-faced babies. Other interaction was limited to bathing, sunbathing, and playing for a total of an hour and a half. The rest of the day was for sleep. Did breastfed babies read the booklet? Obviously not, because they didn't conform to the author's ideas! Hundreds of thousands of mothers gave up breastfeeding when they and their babies were miserable because their breasts didn't make enough milk with only five feeds a day.

Once you're settled at home, maybe your baby's days will be more like these:

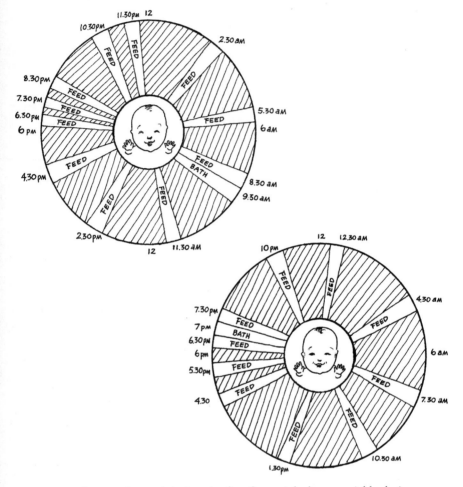

Feeding on demand during the first forty-eight hours quickly drains the thick colostrum, builds your milk production, gives you a chance to learn your baby's feeding cues, and allows your baby plenty of chances to practice this new skill. It also sets the pattern for feeding once your mature milk comes in.

There's much to learn in the first few days after your baby arrives. If you understand the importance of the first feed and learn all you can about your baby's patterns and needs, the easier breastfeeding will be down the road. But that doesn't mean your breastfeeding experience is doomed if all isn't perfect after birth, which is what we'll discuss in the next chapter.

Chapter 4

SPECIAL CONCERNS ABOUT THE FIRST FEED

While it's terrific if your baby can have unrestricted skin-to-skin contact, quickly find your breast, and latch on her own for her first feed, the hours after birth don't always unfold that way. There are a number of reasons why mothers and babies have difficulties or are unable to breastfeed during the first hours, days, or even weeks after birth. If you find yourself in one of these situations, it doesn't mean you can't breastfeed. It just means you'll need to take special steps to get breastfeeding off to the best start you can. This chapter features some common questions new mothers have about the first feed.

What If My Baby Doesn't Feed Right Away at Birth?

Your baby may not want to feed in the first hour after birth, but she'll love skin-to-skin contact with you. Often there's no reason for not sucking—she may just want to rest, keep warm against your skin, and look at you. She's been on a long journey and needs time to adjust, so just enjoy this special time together, which will be etched into your memory forever. If you think she needs some extra guidance, then you might like to try the cross cradle hold (see page 37), but don't put your hand on her head or have your caregiver or nurse do so either.

Just a little note to tell you how blessed I am—Ollie is the perfect feeder after all the nipple problems, expressing, and bottle-feeding I had with his big sister, Caroline. Ollie arrived weighing nine pounds. His first feed about one hour after birth was just a bit of a nuzzle as he was very sleepy. About one hour later, though—wow—give it to me now, Mom! Absolutely enthusiastic! So I latched him on myself right from the second feed and never had any assistance in that regard from then on. He just knew what he was doing.

—Lisa

What If I Have Pain Medication during Labor?

Sometimes babies won't suck because they're sleepy from the pain medications their mothers had during labor. If you have medications during labor, they will affect your baby's normal feeding reflexes for quite a long period. Research shows that when babies stay in skin-to-skin contact after a medicated labor, especially when Demerol (also called Pethidine) is used, they will suck eventually. If they're separated from their mothers even just for weighing and dressing, they don't know how to suck when they're returned to their mothers.[1]

If you have an epidural anesthetic during labor, skin-to-skin contact is vitally important. In natural labor the body releases large amounts of oxytocin during the Fergusson reflex or the urge to push, but an epidural blocks this. (The urge to push and oxytocin release are also of course blocked with a cesarean as well. For more on cesareans, see the next section.) If you have a long period of uninterrupted skin-to-skin time after birth, your baby will help you release lots of oxytocin by massaging your breasts with her hands and fists and the top of your uterus with her feet.

As you can see, the use of medications during labor does affect breastfeeding. Natural labor creates the best conditions for breastfeeding, but if you want or need medication, you can reduce its negative effects by making sure you have skin-to-skin contact with your baby until she attempts to feed.

How Will Having a Cesarean Affect Breastfeeding?

If you have a cesarean, you'll receive either an epidural or spinal anesthetic (in which case you'll be fully conscious when your baby is born) or a general anesthetic (in which case you'll be unconscious). As with other labor medications, these anesthetics will affect you and your baby. However, that doesn't mean you won't be able to breastfeed within the first hour after the birth. You'll need to arrange for skin-to-skin contact with your baby as soon as possible after the operation, usually in the recovery room. Many mothers who've had multiple cesareans have experienced fewer breastfeeding difficulties when they've had skin-to-skin contact immediately after a cesarean than when they'd been separated from their babies.

For many years, doctors told women who had cesareans that their breasts would fill with mature milk much later than if they had had vaginal deliveries. They did have more breastfeeding difficulties than women with vaginal deliveries, but it was more a result of hospital postpartum practices than cesareans themselves. Milk production begins when the mother delivers her placenta or when the doctor extracts it during a cesarean. Although a mother who has a cesarean doesn't have the push urge and oxytocin release, if she has skin-to-skin contact for nipple stimulation, she won't have any more breastfeeding problems than a mother who has had a vaginal birth.

In some hospitals, if both mother and baby are doing well, the baby is placed on the mother's chest underneath the sterile drapes while the obstetrician stitches up the mother. But because immediate skin-to-skin contact after a cesarean doesn't automatically happen in all hospitals, it's a good idea to speak to the hospital staff about their policy if you know you'll be having a cesarean. You may even want to write a request like the one found on the next page.

Dear Hospital Staff,

I'm looking forward to having my next baby at your hospital soon. Our first baby was born during the night by emergency cesarean twenty-six months ago in another city. I was lucky to have a labor and delivery nurse stay with me in the operating and recovery rooms, and she made sure I had skin-to-skin contact with my daughter as soon as we got to the recovery room. The nurse was very helpful and made sure our daughter was well positioned so I could help her latch. She fed well, and we had a lovely problem-free breastfeeding experience for more than twelve months.

My experience, however, seems to be very different from most women's. I've spoken to a number of women who had scheduled cesareans and then had terrible breastfeeding problems. They didn't have nurses with them in the recovery room and didn't have skin-to-skin contact with their babies there. In fact, they weren't offered skin-to-skin contact at all.

As I'm having a scheduled cesarean this time, I'm writing to learn about specific hospital policy on having a nurse stay with me and my baby. Your staff told me it will depend on how many births are happening at the same time. I've discussed this with my obstetrician, and he suggested I write to you to request that a qualified staff member (nurse, midwife, lactation consultant, or doula) be on site to help me and my baby in the recovery room. Also, could you let me know your policy on early skin-to-skin contact both in the recovery room and in the ward? I would like this contact with my baby as soon as possible to ensure breastfeeding starts off right.

Sincerely,
Bronwyn H.

Things to Do

If you know you're having a cesarean, make an appointment with your caregiver or lactation consultant so you can prepare in these ways:

✔ Watch the video *Mother and Baby...The First Week.*

✔ Learn more about the type of anesthetic you'll have and how it'll affect your desire to breast-feed your baby as soon as possible after birth.

✔ Learn practical positions, such as the football hold (with your baby on a pillow under your arm and her feet behind you) to reduce the weight on your incision in the early days after your cesarean.

What If Hospital Policy Doesn't Allow Me to Have the Breastfeeding Experience I Want?

Around the world, women are struggling to have their birth rights—and rites—return to normal. If you feel strongly about how you'd like your labor, birth, and postpartum period to occur, then research the policies at your local hospital(s) and/or birth center(s). Medicine is big business, and it's interesting to watch the changes that happen when women "vote with their feet" and birth where policies support their wishes.

If you don't have a choice about your birth site, you can respectfully question or request exceptions to policies that trouble you. Remember that policies aren't laws, and that no one can force you to submit yourself or your baby to treatment you believe is not in your best interest. And it's illegal for a hospital to turn away a woman in active labor—so you can't be refused care for "making waves."

If you feel very uncomfortable about making waves, then do the best you can with the policies of your local hospital. If policy states babies must be taken immediately for observation, weighing, and testing, then begin skin-to-skin contact as soon as your baby returns and keep in mind that she may not know how to latch right away. If policy states you must leave the baby to clean up or shower, leave the baby skin-to-skin with your partner.

If your mother breastfed you, she may have told you that you were taken away to the nursery for hours or even days, but you still learned how to breastfeed. She's right: Under perfect conditions, babies *feed instinctively* that first time. But when conditions aren't perfect, babies *learn how to breastfeed* whenever that first feed happens, and learning takes time, patience, and support.

What If I Have Inverted Nipples?

Inverted nipples are nipples that shyly turn in instead of out when they or the areola are touched. There are many recommendations floating about for treating inverted nipples during pregnancy in hopes of making latching easier once the baby begins breastfeeding, but none has proven very helpful. If you have inverted nipples, the main thing you need to do is ensure skin-to-skin contact until the first breastfeed. If your baby is alert at this time, she may latch. If not, you may need to hand-express your colostrum the first day and then pump the next day. You can spoon-feed the colostrum to your baby (see page 97), but she'll still need lots of skin contact to calm her because of the lack of sucking. As soon as you can express at least an ounce, you can start using nipple shields (see pages 107–108) to help draw out your nipples.

Before they even give birth, some mothers with inverted nipples collect colostrum and freeze it in case their babies don't latch right away. This exercise is especially recommended for women who have insulin-dependent diabetes mellitus or hormone-related fertility problems, or women who had low milk supply in the early weeks with a previous baby. You will need to ask your caregiver for some syringes to store your precious drops of colostrum.

Here's how to express and store colostrum during pregnancy:

1. Starting at 34 weeks of pregnancy, hand-express (see pages 20–21) after showering each day, when your breasts are warm and your hands are clean.
2. Use a teaspoon-size syringe to collect the drops of colostrum as you express. Put the syringe in a safe place in the fridge after each use over the next forty-eight hours. If you have a big flow of colostrum, you may

find it easier to express into a small, clean (washed in hot soapy water and rinsed) glass or spoon and then collect it with the syringe from there.

3. After two days or when the syringe is full, put it in a zip-lock bag in the freezer. Use a fresh syringe the next day.

4. If you'll be birthing in a hospital, let your caregiver know you'll be bringing frozen colostrum to your birth. Visit the hospital and find out where you can store the colostrum when you arrive in labor.

5. Make sure your caregiver and hospital staff know you want uninterrupted skin-to-skin contact with your new baby and that you have your colostrum in the freezer in case she doesn't latch and feed.

6. If your baby doesn't latch, you can thaw some of your frozen milk to feed her, and when she's settled, you can express. You'll need to express each time your baby doesn't latch to stimulate your supply.

What If I Have to Express Instead of Breastfeed?

Sometimes babies aren't able or ready to breastfeed for some time after birth. This may happen when a baby needs surgery, has a serious health condition, or is premature. You'll learn more about these situations in the following sections, but one requirement they all share is that the mother must express her colostrum and milk until her baby is ready to feed from the breast. Breastmilk is important for all babies, but it's especially important for the health and recovery of babies with special needs. If your baby has been diagnosed during pregnancy with a special condition and you know in advance that you'll need to express, now's the time to learn all you can so you're ready for this commitment. Even if you don't expect your baby to have any problems, it's still helpful to learn about expressing so you'll be prepared in case an unexpected issue arises after the birth.

When you express, it's important to frequently "tell" your breasts they need to make milk. Your breasts need to learn the pattern of frequent filling and emptying, just as they would if you were feeding your baby at your breast. The more milk you express, the more you'll make. When she feeds at the breast, your baby's feeding pattern prompts and builds your supply, but special-needs babies often stay at the hospital full-time during the early days and weeks. You'll need to prompt your breasts yourself. Your caregiver or lactation consultant may tell you to express every two, three, or four hours—which probably sounds like a lot of clock-watching. The easiest way to organize your schedule during the day is by thinking, "Whenever I grab a bite to eat, that's a good time to express my baby's food." This means you'll express:

- before breakfast
- at your late-morning snack
- at lunchtime
- at your afternoon snack
- after dinner
- at your bedtime snack

In addition to these expressing times, you'll also need to express twice overnight. (See page 57.)

If you're the type who doesn't normally eat between meals, get into the habit by always carrying fruit, a granola bar, or some other quick, healthy snack in your purse or bag or by keeping them in sight on the counter at home. Having easy access to food will help you remember to eat more often. Eating light snacks between meals not only reminds you to express, but it also fuels your body so you can make that wonderful milk.

If you were breastfeeding your baby, her feeding patterns and cues would train your body to release oxytocin and let down milk. You'll need to create your own "feeding pattern" when getting ready to express. Here's a helpful routine:

1. Find a comfortable chair. If you're at the hospital, sit close to your baby. If you're at home, sit in your favorite room, perhaps your baby's room if she has one.
2. Eat a couple of whole, large strawberries (which stimulate your inner lips and contain phenylethylamines that encourage oxytocin release) or enjoy a passionate kiss to help increase oxytocin levels. (Your partner will be pleased to learn kissing is important to the baby's survival!)
3. Play relaxing music—the same tune each time.
4. Take a few swallows of a drink and rub your wet tongue around the inside of your lips.
5. Smell a cloth, receiving blanket, or piece of clothing that's been with your baby. (Some mothers place small, clean cloths under their babies' heads during their hospital visits and take the cloths with them when they express. Likewise, they place small cloths in their bras and put

them under their babies' heads when they leave so the babies know the smell of their milk.)

6. Take a few deep breaths.
7. Think of a calming scene, such as a flowing river.
8. Look at a photo of your baby while you express.

Once your breasts fill with mature milk, your caregiver may suggest expressing for ten minutes on each breast, but you may find it easier and more productive to change sides whenever your flow slows down. Some mothers swap sides every two or three minutes for fifteen minutes, take a break to have a snack or put in a load of laundry, and then do a few more minutes on each breast. Other mothers build an over-abundant supply and only need to express one side each time. The most efficient option is to use an electric double-pumping system so you can express both breasts at the same time. This speeds up pumping sessions and builds your supply faster.

Nighttime expressing is also important. Prolactin, the milk-making hormone, is highest at night, so expressing at that time helps build your milk supply. If you're expressing regularly throughout the day and evening, your breasts will probably wake you in the middle of the night and the early morning because they're overfull. That will give you eight expressions in twenty-four hours, which is probably the number of feeds you'd have with your baby. If you're finding it difficult to build up a good supply during the day, then you'll need to set an alarm to express in the middle of the night and the early morning until your supply is abundant enough to wake you on its own. You may think expressing at night will be tiring, but it can be a pleasant, quiet, dreamy time. Express for a short time on each breast. The hormones will make you drowsy, so you'll easily go back to sleep. Remembering that you'd be up during the night with your baby if she were at home will help you keep this task in perspective.

Collecting and Storing Expressed Milk

Always wash your hands before setting up your pump or before starting your hand-expressing. Before you first use a pump or any storage container—such as bottles or cups with tight caps—wash them in hot, soapy water and then rinse and sterilize them in boiling water on the stove or in a home sterilizing kit. If your baby is still in hospital, then follow the hospital's cleaning and sterilizing policy. When your baby is home from hospital, you won't need to sterilize each time. For daily use, thoroughly rinse the equipment in cold water; wash them in hot, soapy water; rinse; and store them in a clean place. Some mothers also like to sterilize regularly. Breastmilk can absorb smells from the container or fridge, so be sure to store it in a clean, airtight container.

Here are some guidelines for storing and using expressed milk:

- Freshly expressed milk can be kept at room temperature (66°F–75°F or 19°C–24°C) for ten hours or in an insulated cooler for twenty-four hours.
- Freshly expressed milk can be stored at the back of a fridge for eight days.
- Thawed milk can be stored at the back of a fridge for twenty-four hours—don't refreeze thawed milk.
- Frozen milk can be stored in a deep freezer at 0°F for up to six to twelve months.
- Frozen milk can be stored in an upright or cyclic-defrost freezer for three to six months.

You may like to freeze your expressed milk in a clean ice-cube tray. The tray should be covered with plastic, and as soon as the cubes are frozen, they should be stored in a sealable plastic bag labeled with the date. Be sure the cubes stay frozen. If your milk thaws a little and then refreezes, the fat cells may burst, and the taste will be unpleasant for your baby. To thaw the cubes you can either put them in a sterile bottle in the fridge and allow them to thaw slowly or put them in a clean or sterilized bottle, then place the bottle in a container of warm (not boiling) water. Thawed milk needs to be used within twenty-four hours and any unused milk should be discarded. Gently move the bottle from side to side as the milk thaws to keep it mixed. Do not thaw or warm milk in the microwave. Microwaves heat unevenly—the milk in the middle of the container will boil before the rest has fully heated. This diminishes the amounts of immune substances, vitamin C, and long-chain polyunsaturated fatty acids in the milk. Microwaved milk can also contain hot spots that may burn your baby.

What If I Can't Breastfeed after Birth?

Rarely is a mother's inability to feed or have contact with her baby after birth due to her own health condition. Even if you've had a long and tiring labor, you can still rest with your baby on your chest so you don't miss out on the important skin-to-skin contact. Many new mothers think they need to send their babies to the nursery in order to rest, but actually, most women rest easier with their babies close to them.

However, sometimes the first feed is delayed due to the mother's condition, such as when she has high blood pressure. If this is the case with you, you'll need to be in a quiet environment with very little stimulation so you can recover after birth. It's extremely important to listen to your caregiver about when you can have skin-to-skin contact and feed your baby or express your milk once your condition improves.

Your body will begin making milk once you deliver your placenta even if you don't breastfeed or express right away. But the earlier you have skin-to-skin contact and either breastfeed or express, the fewer difficulties you'll have. If you're unable to breastfeed for some time, it's very helpful to express every two hours when you're awake to increase your prolactin levels and therefore your milk supply. Even if you're unconscious, critically ill, or seriously injured from a car accident, your breasts will continue to make milk. Many women on life support have been grateful to wake up and find they're still able to breastfeed because their partners or families had asked caregivers to express their milk with electric pumps. Being able to breastfeed and having that special contact with their babies gives these women a great incentive to recover quickly.

What If My Baby Needs Surgery or Intensive Care after Birth?

Babies requiring surgery or intensive care soon after birth often don't feed or even have contact with their mothers right away. (For information about premature babies who need special care, see pages 63–66.) Although you increase your risk of breastfeeding difficulties the longer you wait for skin-to-skin contact and the first feed, if your baby needs surgery, you can overcome these setbacks with help and encouragement.

♥ Things to Do

If you know your baby will require intensive care or surgery for a condition diagnosed by ultrasound or some other screening during pregnancy, you'll want to:

✔ Ask your caregiver, lactation consultant, or local breast-feeding support group about hand-expressing (see pages 20–21), as you'll need to do this for the precious drops of colostrum over the first forty-eight hours, and about continuing to express once your breasts fill with mature milk (see pages 55–58).

✔ Make arrangements to visit the neonatal intensive care nursery where your baby will be after the birth.

✔ Buy a diary to record what happens each day while your baby is in the hospital. (Nurses and visitors can write in it when you're not with your baby.)

✔ Contact other families who've had a baby with the same problem or condition through a local, national, or international support group.

As soon as your baby is able to ingest milk, a stomach tube will feed your expressed milk to her. It's therefore important to keep up with expressing, even if you need to freeze your milk until she's ready to have it. To ensure that your baby has your lovely sensory input during recovery, sit as close as possible so she knows your face and scent and is calmed by your presence. As your baby improves after the surgery, it's a good idea to ask about kangaroo care (see pages 64–66), as this is very calming for babies who have had many medical procedures.

As soon as your baby's well enough to have some milk by mouth, she can go to the breast. Like mothers with premature babies, you'll need to express most of the milk out of your breast before these early feeds because she'll be learning to coordinate sucking, swallowing, and breathing and won't be ready for the fast flow of milk in a full feed (see pages 65–66).

"Are you going to feed your baby?" my midwife asked. "Nuzzle her to your breast."

"I don't think so," I replied, not understanding at that moment the significance of my answer. I had nursed my other babies soon after they were born. Why did I not want to offer Hannah the comfort of my breast?

The answer dawned on me some days later while sitting in intensive care. I must have known—a maternal instinct—that she could not feed because she would have drowned in my milk. My daughter was born with a congenital abnormality: laryngotracheoesophageal cleft, which is a rare complication of esophageal atresia. Rather than two tubes, a trachea and an esophagus, she had only one, and that complicated her breathing and feeding.

The delay in feeding allowed us a special time to bond—a time of touching, loving, and sharing. When Hannah was nearly a day old, I finally attempted to feed her. She refused a number of times but finally latched onto my breast. I could hear her gulp, and I watched her lose her pink color and turn a dusky blue.

She was admitted to the neonatal intensive care unit, and I was introduced to what would become my commitment, my part of the teamwork: expressing milk she'd receive from a feeding tube in her stomach. It had always been my intention to breastfeed, and expressing gave me an opportunity to be closely involved with her care. Little did I know then that I would be expressing for nearly eighteen months.

—Elizabeth

Sue's Comment: Elizabeth's love and strength as well as her milk have brought Hannah through many operations and difficulties. She couldn't eat solid food until she was seven years old, and when she first went to school, the teachers needed to feed her through a tube into her stomach. Now Hannah is nine, and she's an absolutely delightful child who's working hard at school and has lots of friends. Her survival is due to the power of love and, I suspect, a hundred gallons or more of her mother's expressed milk.

A Baby with a Cleft Lip and/or Cleft Palate

Occurring in one out of every seven hundred births, cleft lip and cleft palate are two of the most common abnormal developments seen at birth, but they're completely repairable. If your baby has a cleft lip and/or cleft palate, she'll need surgery, but it shouldn't prevent you from breastfeeding or at least having a breast experience in the first hours after birth. Breastfeeding can continue for some babies, particularly if they have only a cleft lip, but other babies, particularly those with a large cleft palate, will receive their main nutrition via a tube through the nose into the stomach or from a special feeder.

Positioning a baby with a cleft is quite different than positioning other babies. If your baby has a cleft, she'll need to sit up fairly straight at the breast, perhaps on a cushion at your side. Always face her in the same direction so you can close off the cleft with your fingers and your breast. For example, if she has a cleft on the right side of her lip, use the cradle hold when she feeds on your left breast and the football hold with her on a cushion when she feeds on your right. This way, you can bunch your breast up into the palate and make a seal (for the cradle hold, press your left breast at three o'clock with your right middle finger and for the football hold, press your right breast with your left thumb at three o'clock). Because it won't be a perfect seal, she'll often swallow a lot of air and may need to burp frequently during feeds.

You may be able to use a nipple shield (see pages 107–108) with a supplementer (see pages 76–78) taped behind the shield to feed at the breast. This has many advantages for you both—it slows down the milk flow so your baby can cope with it, it allows the beautiful contact that normally happens with breastfeeding, and it ensures adequate nutrition.

If the cleft is diagnosed during pregnancy, you may decide, after discussion with your caregiver, to express colostrum from the thirty-fourth week of pregnancy onward. Colostrum can be collected in special syringes and be frozen (see pages 54–55). This colostrum can then be given to your baby in the first few days to prevent inner ear problems that can be caused by giving formula to your baby at this time. Inner ear infections are one of the most common illnesses in babies with clefts because their eustachian tubes, the tubes between the throat and the ears, are usually shortened.

What If My Baby Has Down Syndrome?

Babies with Down syndrome or other low-muscle-tone conditions have as much skill at the first feed as other babies, unless they have other medical issues, such as heart problems. In fact, they can sometimes feed with more skill. If your baby has Down syndrome, you'll find that her tongue often lolls out of her mouth. This is a real advantage for the first feed because your baby will lick well and find your breast easily.

Breastmilk and sucking will be very important for your baby. In the past, most mothers were discouraged from breastfeeding babies with Down syndrome, and their babies tended to suffer from ear, throat, chest, and bowel infections; constipation; vomiting after feeds; obesity; and skin disorders. Because your baby can easily digest your breastmilk, she'll be less likely to vomit or become constipated. In addition, the long-chain polyunsaturated fatty acids in your breastmilk will lead to optimal brain and retina development, and they'll reduce the chance of skin disorders. The antibodies in your breastmilk will also help protect your baby against bowel, chest, and ear infections as well as reduce the severity of any allergies.

When babies bottle-feed, they use only jaw and tongue muscles; when babies breastfeed, they use all their facial muscles. Breastfeeding will strengthen the muscles your baby uses to control her tongue thrust and drooling. The distinctive Down syndrome facial shape will also change as she develops a fat pad in the masseter muscles of her cheeks, which will make her cheekbones appear higher and her face much plumper. This muscle development will help her eat solids and talk earlier than similar babies who have not been breastfed. Her physical development—being able to roll over, crawl, and walk—will be less delayed as well because she won't be as obese as formula-fed babies with Down syndrome.

What If My Baby Is Premature?

Caregivers usually need to take premature babies to the neonatal intensive care nursery within a few minutes of their birth. If your baby is premature but has a good Apgar score—an assessment of her color, breathing, heart rate, muscle tone, and reflexes at birth—her caregiver may encourage you to have a quick cuddle or at least look at your baby before taking her to the nursery. However, some premature babies are not just small but very sick, and it's necessary for them to go to the nursery almost immediately.

If this happens with your baby, put your energy into expressing your milk (see pages 55–58), which your baby will receive as soon as tube feedings are allowed. This is the most positive and practical thing you can do for your tiny, beautiful child. Milk made for premature babies is different from milk made for full-term babies. Your body is clever enough to know that your baby needs more protein and also more epidermal growth factor (EGF), a form of protein that promotes cell growth. EGF is in your amniotic fluid, and if your baby is born early, she'll receive it in your milk. This means she can keep up with the growth and development that would have occurred if she hadn't been born early. EGF is particularly important for the growth of her immature esophagus, stomach, and intestines.

> Premature babies need eye and mouth cleanings every four hours. You might want to suggest that your baby's caregivers first use your colostrum and then your milk for this purpose. Colostrum promotes normal esophagus development, and eye infections have been effectively treated for many years with breastmilk.[2]

Kangaroo Care

When your baby is premature, you may hear the old warning, "Don't handle your baby too much because she won't gain weight," but many studies since 1985 have disproved this belief. Even premature and sick babies now come out of their incubators for special skin-to-skin contact called kangaroo care. The babies, dressed only in diapers, are placed inside their parents' clothing, much like baby kangaroos in their mothers' pouches. In as little as thirty-five minutes a day, kangaroo care can make many improvements in your baby's health: She'll experience fewer temperature changes than in the incubator, higher oxygen levels, less change in her heart and breathing rates, less initial weight loss, quicker weight gain, and less crying. Most importantly, it'll help you produce larger amounts of breastmilk and breastfeed for a longer period over the months and years ahead.

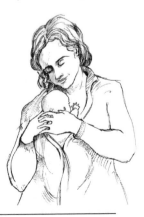

I remember sitting in the nursery during the first few days, looking at Rosie through the side of her hospital bassinet, and I didn't feel she was mine. But once we started kangaroo care, I didn't just feel body-to-body closer, I really felt that I knew her and that she remembered me. One of the things she loved was for me to hold her hand as she fell asleep. We still kanga quite a bit at home even though she's quite big now and has nearly doubled her birth weight—it must be all that lovely breastmilk!

—Megan

As your baby's health improves, you can begin breastfeeding. Although babies learn how to breastfeed most easily when left skin-to-skin with their mothers at birth, it doesn't mean you won't be able to breastfeed your premature baby. It just means that instead of her latching on to your breast and sucking instinctively, you'll need to teach her how to do it.

Full-term babies drink about one-half to one teaspoon of thick, concentrated colostrum at each feed in the first few days. This small amount of fluid gives babies a few days to learn how to suck, swallow, and breathe in an easy sequence. It's a very important learning time. As babies slowly learn this skill over the next ten to twenty feeds, their swallowing rates increase, and so does the amount of milk their mothers make. After that point, they can then easily cope with six or seven sucks and swallows to each breath.

Your tiny baby needs this learning time, too, but as the research of Indira Narayanan and others has shown, this is easier on an emptied breast. Your premature baby may cough, sputter, and become frightened by the rush of milk from a full breast. So just after you express, let her lick, nuzzle, and start to suckle. Like a full-term baby, she may need ten to twenty practices to learn to suck, swallow, and breathe before she's ready to feed from a full breast. These first few times your baby is at the breast won't be for feeding but for the sensory joy of your smell, the softness of your breast, and the sweet taste of your milk as she licks it off your nipple. This learning time will make future breastfeeds easy and pleasurable for you both.

As your baby makes some sucking movements over the next few days, you can help her understand the rhythm of feeding by squeezing your breast behind the areola and expressing the milk into her mouth at the rate of one squeeze per second. It helps to hold her close with her feet at the same level as her head and to be in a room with soft lights and quiet music. Music with sixty to seventy beats per minute, such as baroque or country, mimics a heartbeat and encourages the correct sucking pattern of one suck per second. Before long, your premature baby will be able to breastfeed as well as a full-term baby.

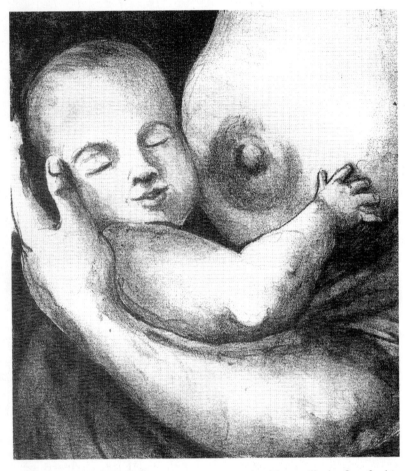

Whether your baby is full-term or premature, healthy or ill, the first feed is important no matter when it happens. While not all babies have an opportunity to feed instinctively under the perfect conditions right after birth, all babies—and mothers—learn how to breastfeed in time. Whenever you're able to bring you baby home, you can continue this important education there.

Chapter 5
BRINGING YOUR BABY HOME

When mothers stayed in the hospital longer than they do now, they had time to get a baby-care education from their doctors and nurses. Nowadays, most women leave the hospital within forty-eight hours, and they still have a lot to learn about their babies and breastfeeding.

We now understand from Barbara Attrill's research that once her baby arrives, a mother is "oriented to her own physical and emotional needs" as she takes in the enormous changes. During this "taking in" period she needs to tell the story of her labor and birth many times and usually feels vague, disorganized, and unable to absorb information. Learning how to breastfeed and care for a new baby can be difficult under these conditions. This is why it's important to learn as much as possible about breastfeeding and parenting during pregnancy and why it's important to have good support after the baby is born.

Your baby dramatically changes your lifestyle. This tiny person will, ironically, consume huge amounts of your time and your emotional and physical energy. He'll breastfeed eight to twelve times in twenty-four hours, taking forty-five to sixty minutes for each feed, including diaper changing and cuddles. Added up, feeding will take at least eight hours each day. It's natural to wonder if your baby is getting enough milk at this time, so you need to watch carefully for signs that he's thriving (see page 71). Learning how to cope with sleepless nights is also a big part of this early period. Egyptian hieroglyphics about family life have revealed that their babies cried from dusk until dead of night. Well, thousands of years later, babies are still behaving the same way!

Many people refer to the first weeks after birth as the "fourth trimester." Much like each trimester of pregnancy, the postpartum trimester is a time when both you and the baby grow and change a lot. Mothering doesn't always come naturally and neither does breastfeeding, so be patient as you develop these new skills.

Chapter 5

When Your Milk Comes In

After forty-eight hours, your colostrum will begin changing into mature milk. During this change, you'll go from making two to four ounces of colostrum on the second day to eighteen to twenty-eight ounces of milk during the fifth day. This milk is higher in lactose, fat, and casein proteins than colostrum but lower in whey proteins (antibodies). Many first-time mothers describe their milk coming in as a tightening of the chest and breasts that makes them take a few deep breaths in wonder at this sudden change in their bodies. Other mothers don't recognize the change until they hear their babies swallowing much more at a feed.

Your baby will feed eight to twelve times each day, and his time at the breast may be as little as fifteen to twenty minutes or as much as thirty to forty-five minutes, depending on your milk flow, how vigorously your baby feeds, and whether he drinks from one or both breasts. When your colostrum first changes to milk, your baby may be happy to finish the first breast but too full to take the second. Many babies can get plenty of milk from one breast, and the more your baby drains one breast, the creamier the milk becomes. This is because hind milk (which flows as your breast starts to drain) is higher in fat than fore milk (which flows when your baby first latches on to the breast). If you use both breasts at each feed when your supply is too much for his appetite, then your baby will get more lower-fat milk (fore milk), and he may be unsettled and miserable even though he has plenty of wet and soiled diapers. Offering one breast at each feed leaves him satisfied without overfilling his tummy. Eventually, your baby will want both breasts at most or all feeds. For now, one breast will likely be enough because you probably make more milk than your baby needs. In essence, your breasts make lots of milk because they don't "know" your baby's birth weight and they therefore don't know how much he needs. Making lots of milk ensures he'll have enough no matter how big he is. Your supply will most likely settle down after a couple of days, but for some mothers it takes a couple of weeks or even months. At that point, most babies will want both breasts at each feed, but some babies will always be satisfied with just one breast.

Whether he feeds from one or both breasts at a feeding, hopefully your baby has had unrestricted feeding from both breasts over the past few days. Equal drainage and long periods of sucking over twenty-four hours may prevent your breasts from becoming engorged, as your thick colostrum will have been removed. This will let your mature milk flow easily once your breasts fill.

Venous Engorgement

In order for your breasts to make lots of milk, you need a good supply of blood to bring them all the necessary nutrients. You'll find lots of veins showing on your chest and breasts during the third and fourth day. When this increase in blood supply occurs, your breast tissue may swell, which causes venous engorgement. This happens when the arteries bring lots of blood to the breasts but the veins take it away too slowly.

If this happens, here are some tips to try:

- Express a little milk to soften the areola before your baby latches.
- Drain the first breast before offering the second.
- If your baby feeds on only one breast, offer the other at the next feed.
- The easiest way to overcome breast engorgement is to put something cool on your breasts, such as ice packs. Cover the packs with cloths, and apply them for only ten minutes each hour. Longer ice application may damage the blood circulation in your breasts in the long term. The coolness will constrict or tighten the blood vessels. After about ten minutes the blood vessels will dilate, or enlarge. This takes the blood away from the breasts quickly, and the swelling will gradually subside over the next forty-eight hours.
- In the shower, turn your breasts away from the hot water because the relaxing warmth will bring extra blood flow to your breasts and increase the swelling. Also, the heat will make your breasts leak, which may lead to milk engorgement (see next section) because your breasts will respond to the leak by making even more milk.

Milk Engorgement

While milk engorgement was common in the days when mothers and babies were on strict feeding schedules and separated in hospitals, it's a fairly rare condition in these days of rooming-in and feeding on demand. It can occur, however, if you force a feeding schedule with only five minutes on each breast and no night feeds. It can also happen if you have a huge oversupply of milk in the first four days that your baby can't possibly drain. This may be due to a hormonal disease that makes your body produce too much prolactin. If you've never been diagnosed with this condition, milk engorgement may be your first sign of it, so talk to your caregiver.

If you experience milk engorgement, your breasts will be abnormally full and enlarged and possibly so heavy you can hardly get out of bed. When your breasts are this full, your nipples may be compressed (flattened) and painful, and your baby can't latch easily. Poor latching means your baby can't drain your breast, but the milk he has drunk is replaced and your breasts become abnormally full again. It's vitally important that your breasts don't get warm in the shower, because that'll bring extra blood and oxytocin. This can start a letdown of milk. The letdown sends the milk from the milk sacs into the ducts for removal by your baby, but there's no baby in the shower to drink it! A small amount of milk may leak from your nipples, but most of it will sit in your ducts and overfill your breasts. The swelling will also increase as the milk sacs replace the milk that has flowed into the ducts.

If you experience milk engorgement, use all the suggestions on page 69 for relieving venous engorgement. Then do the following *only for the next two feeds*:
- Express one to two ounces of milk from the breast you're going to feed from. As soon as you have expressed, feed your baby on this breast only. Apply ice packs to both breasts after the feed.
- Right before the next feed, express one to two ounces of milk from the other breast, and feed your baby from that breast only. Again, apply cold packs to both breasts at the end of the feed.

If necessary at the following feeds, express only a small amount of milk to soften your areola, and feed only on one breast per feed (alternating breasts with each feed) until your milk supply has settled down.

Knowing Your Baby Is Getting Enough Milk

During the first forty-eight hours after birth, you started to learn your baby's feeding cues so you could feed him according to his own needs and not a forced schedule. As you continue this at home and your baby drinks more and more of your mature milk, you may still wonder if he's getting enough. You, like many breastfeeding mothers, may find this to be one of the first tests of your confidence. You may ask yourself, "Is my milk really flowing, and how much does my baby need to drink?"

Carefully watch for a number of signs during each feed to tell if your milk is flowing and your baby is getting enough to drink:

- You'll become thirsty.
- You may perspire.
- You may have milk dripping from your other breast.
- You'll see your baby's ears wiggle as his whole jaw works to suck and swallow.
- You'll hear your baby swallowing. After each suck, he'll rhythmically pause to swallow, and you'll hear either a small sound (as if you said the *cu* sound of *cup* in the back of your throat) or a big gulping sound. If your baby isn't swallowing, you'll see fast sucking and no slight pause or you won't hear the swallowing sound.
- Your baby will detach when he's done and look very blissful and sleepy. Some babies fall asleep at the breast before they finish their feed. If your baby falls asleep at the breast and doesn't detach, detach him by sliding your short-nailed little finger into his mouth to break his suction. Your breast will slide out of his mouth. Wake him by changing his diaper, and then see if he'll feed again.
- Your breast will feel much softer and lighter than it did before the feed.

In addition, check for these other signs that your baby is thriving:

- His stool will change from green-black to green-brown and then to mustard yellow.
- He'll have five to six heavy, wet diapers a day.
- He'll start to regain the weight he lost since birth (see next section), which your caregiver will determine at his first checkup.

Before you read on, you need to know the difference between a "wet" and a "damp" diaper. Using two disposable diapers, pour four tablespoons of water into one diaper and pour one tablespoon into another. Hold a diaper in each hand. The damp diaper (one tablespoon) will feel much lighter than the wet one (four tablespoons).

To get a better feel for how much your baby eats and how many diapers he goes through, you may find it helpful to fill in the worksheet on page 72 for a day or two. This isn't a way to force a feeding schedule on him. It's just a way to see the pattern he has established on his own.

Date_____

Diaper Clocks

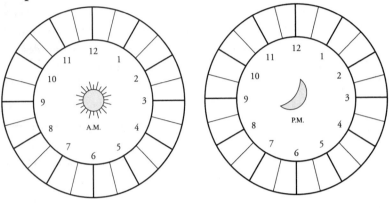

Wet diapers:_____   Poopy diapers:_____

Activity Clocks

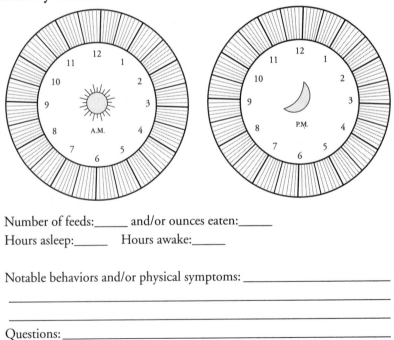

Number of feeds:_____ and/or ounces eaten:_____
Hours asleep:_____   Hours awake:_____

Notable behaviors and/or physical symptoms: _____
_____
_____

Questions: _____
_____
_____
_____

Diaper Clocks

Whenever you change a wet diaper, note the time and write a *W* in the corresponding spot on the rim of the appropriate diaper clock. Whenever you change a poopy diaper, write a *P*. At the end of the day, tally your baby's wet and poopy diapers and write the totals in the spaces provided.

Activity Clocks

Each bar on the activity clocks represents five minutes. Whenever you feed your baby, note the starting and ending times of the feeding and fill in the corresponding bars on the rim of the appropriate activity clock. Write an *R* (for right) or an *L* (for left) next to the feeding to indicate which breast you offered first. With a different-colored pen or pencil, record your baby's sleep periods in the same way. The remaining blank bars represent your baby's awake (nonfeeding) periods. At the end of the day, tally the total number of feeds and the total hours of asleep and awake time in the spaces provided.

Notes and Questions

If you observe any notable behaviors or physical symptoms in your baby, record them in the space provided. For example, you might record a long crying jag, fever, unusual-looking diaper contents, rash, and so on. Similarly, if you think of a question you'd like to ask an expert (for example, your baby's caregiver or a lactation consultant), record it in the space provided.

When Your Baby Needs Immediate Medical Attention

During the first three or four days of life, many changes happen in your baby's body. He will probably lose 5–8 percent of his weight at birth from passing his meconium (early green-black stool) and from normal fluid loss during breathing and sweating. This is normal. The occurrences outlined below, however, are not normal. If you encounter these, you should contact your baby's caregiver.

Urates

As your colostrum changes to milk and your baby drinks more at each feed, he'll flush out the salts (or urates) in his kidneys. You'll see them as a pink-orange, rusty stain in his wet diaper about seventy-two hours after his birth.

If you see urates in his diaper when he's four or five days old, this is abnormal, particularly if he's still passing green-black stools and not feeding lustily. You need to take your baby to his caregiver or the urgent care clinic immediately.

Dehydration

Dehydration occurs when a baby does not get enough milk once the hibernation stage (see page 44) is over. This most often happens when a baby isn't latched well and can't drink enough, if a mother uses a nipple shield (see pages 107–108) when her flow doesn't necessitate it, or when a mother is unable to make sufficient milk because of a hormonal problem or previous breast surgery (see pages 4–6).

If your baby is more than seventy-two hours old, watch for the following signs of dehydration. If you notice these signs, then you need to take your baby to his caregiver or the urgent care clinic immediately.

- Your baby is sleepy and doesn't wake to feed often (at least six feeds every twenty-four hours), or he wakes often to feed, but he just sucks quickly with only a few swallows before falling asleep again at all or most feeds.
- He doesn't swallow frequently and rhythmically in the first five minutes of each feed.

- He cries when you detach him and searches for the breast again, but immediately closes his eyes and goes back to his fast sucking and no swallowing.
- He frowns while sucking at the breast.
- He has "damp" but not "wet" diapers (see page 71).
- He has tiny amounts of black or brown stool.
- His skin and the whites of his eyes grow increasingly jaundiced.
- He has loose folds of skin on his limbs, back, and abdomen.
- You have no change in breast fullness from the beginning to the end of each feed.

One of the things your baby's caregiver will order is extra milk. To express easily during this stressful time, you may want to use an electric pump or rent one from a hospital. The hospital lactation consultant can help you overcome any positioning and latching difficulties and teach you how to use a supplementer (see pages 76–77).

Things to Do

Ask to see the video *Mother and Baby...the First Week*. This video shows urates, yellow skin color, and changes in stool color and provides hints on overcoming breastfeeding difficulties that can lead to health problems for your baby.

Weight-Gain Problems

When thriving on your milk, your baby will gain five to seven ounces each week for the first six to eight weeks. If your baby isn't getting enough milk, he won't gain this much weight or he'll even lose weight. Weight-gain problems often occur when babies drink from only one breast at most or all feeds. Once your milk supply settles after your colostrum changes to mature milk (see page 68), your baby needs to drink from both breasts at each feed. To prevent weight-gain problems from becoming serious, take note of your baby's feeding and diaper patterns. Watch for the following signs:

- Your baby stays on one breast for more than thirty minutes.
- He takes only sleepy sucks with little swallowing for almost all of the feed.
- He's unsettled when you detach him.
- He has only damp diapers (see page 71).

If you see these signs, you may need to frequently swap your baby from one breast to the other during feeds. Swapping breasts means your milk will flow much faster. As your baby begins to feed from your first breast, milk ejections let down milk in your second breast at the same time, and this milk collects in the breast.[1] When your baby switches breasts, the second breast starts off with faster-flowing milk than the first breast did. This is why frequent swapping helps your sleepy baby feed more easily and actively.

While weight-gain problems are very serious, you certainly don't need to buy scales and chart your baby's weight yourself. That's something your baby's caregiver will do at regular checkups. Your great-grandma didn't need scales to know whether her children were doing okay, and neither do you! Between checkups, note the following when you bathe your baby, just as your great-grandmother did with her children:

- Does he have dull eyes?
- Are his mouth and lips dry?
- Does the skin on his body and legs feel saggy as you hold him?
- Are his diapers damp (not wet) (see page 71) and stained yellow?
- Does he sleep for long periods at night?

If you answered yes to the previous questions, your baby needs to see his caregiver as soon as possible.

If your baby isn't thriving, you'll most likely need to:

- Improve his latch with assistance from your lactation consultant.
- Switch from side to side every time he looks sleepy, which may be every five minutes. He may need to go to each breast two or three times per feed. (Remember, your milk will become creamier and flow faster at each change.)
- Wait twenty minutes after the feed, then express for five minutes total with an electric double-pump or five minutes on each breast with an electric single-pump or manual pump.
- Set an alarm to feed your baby during the night if he doesn't wake on his own.
- Monitor his weight twice over the following four days with help from your baby's caregiver.

Using a Supplementer

If your baby has lost more weight at either of the weight checks, his caregiver may suggest you use a supplementer during feeds. A supplementer is a special bottle with a fine tube threaded through the lid. You fill the supplementer with milk and wear it around your neck so it hangs between your breasts. One end of the tube is below the milk level in the supplementer, and you tape the other end to your areola so the opening is at the tip of your nipple. As your baby sucks, he'll drink milk from your breast and also draw milk from the supplementer through the tube. This is an easy way for him to get the extra calories he needs to get his energy back, stay awake, feed properly, and thrive again.

If possible, it's best for the milk in the supplementer to be your expressed breastmilk. However, you may have to consider other options if he needs a full feed before you can express enough or if your supply is low and you can't yet make enough. If this happens, you can either use donated milk from a milk bank (see page 11) or ask your baby's caregiver to prescribe a hypoallergenic formula.

You may feel crushed and even lose confidence in your mothering skills if you need to supplement your breastmilk. Instead, feel good that you were smart and strong enough to get medical help for your baby. With help, the whole situation can be turned around, your breastfeeding can continue, and your baby can return to good health. That's the most important part.

I have just fed Victoria, and while she (temporarily!) nods off I will write to you. Thank you for knowing how much breastfeeding matters to me. Receiving help silenced many a potential critic. I still don't know if she'll ever take a full feed from me, but needing the supplementer isn't as big a deal as it seemed months ago. The most stressful thing through it all was taking her to be weighed—it seemed like a test of my motherhood. Justin decided he would take her to be weighed, and I feel so much less stressed and pressured. I know that what I'm doing for Victoria is natural and right for us both. Ultimately my family will benefit from our perseverance.

—Danielle

(Sue's note: Danielle had a breast reduction, and even after trying all the other options to help her supply—such as improving latching, swapping breasts frequently, and taking medication to increase her supply—the supplementer was necessary.)

I've finally found time to write and let you know what happened to my milk supply. You may remember Andrew was a very placid baby who fed often but for short times during the day and who slept up to ten hours at night at four weeks old. I remember how pleased Michael and I were and how we felt sorry for friends whose babies fed every two or three hours day and night.

You probably also remember how upset I was when the doctor said Andrew was losing weight and that I would need to give him formula after each feed if I wanted to keep on breast-feeding. The supplementer sounded like a good idea, but it was so hard to start with, and setting the alarm at odd hours in the night was much worse than when he wakes us now!

But at the next weigh-in, the tears of joy came fairly quickly when we found out he gained so much. Thank you for helping me get the equipment and for listening. I get quite scared thinking how much weight he lost and how sick he could have been.

—Nicky

Nighttime Feeding

Research has shown that babies receive a third of their nutrition during the night.[2] Knowing this may help you realize that feeding at night is something your baby not only wants to do but also needs to do in order to gain weight and thrive. Getting your baby to sleep through the night should not be a parenting goal or a sign of your "success." This is why so many mothers didn't reach their breastfeeding goals in the past. They were taught that their babies needed eight hours of sleep at night. This simply meant their breasts didn't drain often enough, their milk supply decreased, and their babies didn't gain enough weight, so they weaned.

Remember how often you needed to go to the bathroom during the night when you were pregnant? Your baby would wake you by gently bouncing on your bladder as he moved around during his wakeful times. Are these the same wakeful times your baby has now? Quite possibly they are. Some babies keep to their fetal waking times after they are born, while others develop new patterns.

Bed-Sharing and Cosleeping

Bed-sharing was a cultural norm in most cultures until the Industrial Revolution, when women had to leave their babies to go back to work. As they lost the contraceptive effect of frequent breastfeeding, their fertility increased. This meant there were more mouths to feed, and therefore even more need to work. Some researchers have suggested that during this period parents practiced infanticide and reported it as "overlaying" to suggest they had accidentally rolled onto their babies during sleep. In the hope of preventing the alleged overlaying, some religions began to teach that it was psychologically and morally bad for children to share their parents' bed. The effects of these teachings have survived, and parents today continue to worry about children sharing their bed.[3]

Actually, it's often safer for a baby to share his parents' bed or room than to sleep on his own. Research into sudden infant death syndrome (SIDS) suggests that babies are safer if they share their parents' bedroom, and this is supported in recent policy of the American Academy of Pediatrics.[4] It's now known that putting babies to sleep on their stomachs, using quilts, putting babies on free-flow waterbeds, and parents' smoking or use of alcohol or drugs all increase the likelihood of SIDS.[5] But when parents and babies share a bedroom under safe conditions, it's beneficial. Early findings from ongoing research in the United States show that mother and baby synchronize their breathing when bed-sharing. If the baby's breathing changes, the mother will wake. In many hospitals, mothers and babies are again sharing beds as nurseries disappear.

Some parents want to have their baby in their bedroom but not necessarily in their bed. Cosleeping, as this is called, is easily done by taking off the crib rail and putting the crib beside your bed so its mattress is at the same height as yours. You can then make a continuous mattress by tucking in an extra flat sheet across your bed and into the opposite side of the crib mattress. This allows you easy access to your baby and him easy access to you. Because feeding frequently throughout the day and night is important to maintaining a good milk supply, you may find cosleeping to be the perfect setup. You can wake when your baby first stirs, pick him up, feed him, and put him down again without ever leaving your bed. (If he needs a clean diaper after a feed, you might have to get out of bed, but you don't need to go very far!) Cosleeping also means he'll be in arm's reach if he needs soothing. This is important because until babies are six months old, they have no awareness that somebody is always there to care for them. When your baby is awake and away from body contact, he'll cry for it to return, much as other baby animals do when their mothers move away for a short time.

You'll need to work through your feelings about sharing your bedroom or bed with your baby, but know that it can be quite safe and beneficial. If you do bed-share or cosleep, you can plan to move him into his own room whenever it works best for your family.

Getting Your Baby Back to Sleep

You may have nights when your baby wakes once or twice to feed, then falls blissfully asleep. You may have other nights when it seems your baby refuses to fall asleep even after he's fed.

Knowing your baby's sleep cycle can help you get him back to sleep after nighttime feeds. Your baby has a different sleep cycle than you. Adults have a ninety-minute sleep cycle with 75 percent deep or quiet sleep and 25 percent dream or REM (rapid eye movement) sleep. Your baby has a much shorter cycle of forty-five minutes divided into twenty to twenty-five minutes of both deep sleep and REM sleep. After a feed, your baby will be in REM sleep, and he'll wake very easily because his brain is active. Knowing this, you may find it useful to cuddle him for about twenty minutes after a feed so he'll move into deep sleep and be less likely to wake when you put him to bed. After three months, these sleep cycles will alter, and your baby will find it easier to fall asleep on his own.

Things to Do

If you have trouble getting your baby back to sleep at night, try these tips:

✔ Warm a lightweight receiving blanket against your skin while you're feeding him. As you put him back into his bed, put the wrap under him and tuck it in carefully, like a bottom sheet. Your baby will go to sleep more easily in a place that's warm and smells like you.

✔ Partly feed him before changing his diaper. This is so he doesn't cry, getting hungrier and hungrier, while you change his diaper. The less he cries, the more easily he'll settle after his feed.

✔ Turn on only a dim light (or keep the lights off) while you feed him. Babies don't recognize day from night until about three months, and the darkness or semidarkness may help him learn that nighttime is the time to sleep.

✔ Don't talk to him in a loud voice—chatting is for daytime.

Who Gets Up?: A Hypothetical Tale of Parenthood

Parents who bottle-feed often take turns getting up to feed their babies in the night. Obviously, you're the only one who can feed your baby, and you need to be at least partly awake to do so. Although you and your partner can't take turns feeding, either one of you can get the baby to bring him back to bed for feeding (if you're not bed-sharing). Although it may seem like a good idea to take turns equally, you'll probably discover that every night is a little different, depending on how your and your partner's day has played out. It may not be as easy as "your turn, my turn." Take time to read the following tale starting on page 82 with your partner. In this scenario, the mother is at home with the baby on maternity leave and the partner works outside the home. Decide together who would get up to fetch the baby for each feed.

Sunday

The baby is twelve days old and besides the two evenings when he cried for five hours, he's been reasonably settled. It's Sunday, and you've been to Grandma and Grandpa's for lunch and have arrived home at 5:30 PM. You bathe the baby at 7:00 PM, and he's fed and asleep by 8:15. Instead of going to bed early, you and your partner both decide to stay up and watch a movie. After the movie, you get to sleep at 11:00 PM.

1. The baby wakes at 11:30 PM—who gets up? _____

2. The baby wakes at 2:00 AM—who gets up? _____

3. The baby wakes at 5:30 AM——who gets up? _____

Monday

Your partner goes off to work and has a very busy, stressful day. Even though there's still work to do, your partner manages to leave work a little earlier than usual and rushes home to help you. As for you, you've had a lovely day at home. The baby fed at 9:00 AM, 11:30 AM, and 3:30 PM and went straight back to sleep after each feed, so you got a long afternoon nap. You both go to bed early for your partner's sake after the baby has fed on and off from 5:30 to 8:30 PM.

1. The baby wakes at 11:30 PM—who gets up? _____

2. The baby wakes at 3:00 AM—who gets up? _____

3. The baby wakes at 6:00 AM—who gets up? _____

Tuesday

Your partner goes off to work, feeling particularly chipper and confident about parenthood. You talk at lunchtime, and although the baby has fed every couple hours, he's finally sleeping, so you encourage your partner to go out with friends after work. Your partner arrives home at 7:30 PM to find the house in a mess with wet laundry draped over the kitchen chairs. The baby is crying, and you seem unable to console him. You yourself burst into tears. You hand over the baby, saying you need a shower. As soon as your partner takes over, the baby falls asleep within ten minutes! You come back from the shower and tell the story of the terrible day you've had: The baby fed at 8:30, 10:30, 1:00, and 4:00, and up until your partner came home, the baby cried constantly after a few minutes on the breast every half hour. Your partner cooks a lovely meal, and life looks brighter. The baby wakes, feeds, and settles quickly at 10:00 PM, and then you all go to bed.

1. The baby wakes at 1:00 AM—who gets up?   _____

2. The baby wakes at 4:30 AM—who gets up?   _____

Wednesday

You have a family breakfast at 7:30 AM, and then the baby has a calm day, sleeping for a couple of hours after each feed. Your partner comes home to a much brighter pair than last night. After a pleasant meal, during which the baby has been at the breast, the baby continues to feed on and off until 9:30 PM. You and your partner go to bed early.

1. The baby wakes at 11:30 PM—who gets up?   _____

2. The baby wakes at 2:30 AM—who gets up?   _____

3. The baby wakes at 5:30 AM—who gets up?   _____

As you can see, no two days—or nights—are the same, but I doubt you could say that they ever were, even before you had a baby! Babies' sleeping and eating habits tend to differ every day in the early weeks. The differences from one day to another will take a little time to get used to. Doing the previous exercise will help you see that there's a lot more to consider than "It's your turn!" when someone needs to get the baby for a feed. Talk about how your own days and nights have been going and whether you'd like to handle the nighttime feeds differently.

Getting Yourself Enough Sleep

Sleep is key to your health and well-being, so it's important to get eight hours of sleep every twenty-four hours. Getting up with the baby during the night will no doubt break up your nighttime sleep. Luckily, the oxytocin and prolactin released during each feed will make you tired and help you go back to sleep quickly. Still, you probably won't be able to get all eight hours of sleep at night, so you'll need to make them up at different times throughout the day. It's good to either stay in bed later in the morning or nap in the afternoon. Hopefully, you can plan to do both in the early weeks. Let your support people worry about the laundry or the dishes. Going to bed early is also helpful. It may be tempting to stay up and wait for your baby's late-evening feed, but it's better to be disturbed after an hour's sleep than to lose an hour of sleep waiting for a feed he may not want.

Getting plenty of rest is very important with breastfeeding, especially during those first days at home. As you'll learn in the next chapter, new mothers can encounter many common problems as they learn to breastfeed. Anything you can do to either avoid these problems or quickly overcome them will help you and your baby have a positive, successful breastfeeding experience.

Chapter 6

SOLUTIONS TO COMMON PROBLEMS

A lot can go right with breastfeeding, but sometimes a lot can go wrong. Even if you avoided engorgement when your milk came in (see pages 68–70) and kept your baby from getting dehydrated or having weight problems (see pages 74–78) when you first brought her home, painful nipples, painful breasts, or other problems that complicate breastfeeding may still occur. But rest assured that nearly every problem has a solution, so you can overcome your difficulties and have a successful breastfeeding experience.

Painful Nipples

In the early twentieth century, doctors thought women's nipples weren't tough enough to tolerate babies' sucking. Doctors assumed the solution was to tell pregnant women to "toughen up" their nipples with rough towels, nailbrushes, or methylated spirits each day. (I can imagine your nipples hiding at the thought of this!) Unfortunately, the treatment made painful and bleeding nipples more, not less, common. We now know sore nipples are often symptoms of improper latching and overfull breasts. We also know rough towels and nailbrushes remove natural oils from the skin, causing nipples to become even more cracked and dry. While those harmful methods are no longer in practice, some people suggest using creams and ointments every day to make nipples soft and supple. Many of these products are on the market, but they haven't been shown to prevent sore nipples.[1] Most of them are based on lanolin taken from sheep's wool. As your baby knows you by your smell, I'm sure you don't want her to mistake you for a sheep! To prevent or cure painful nipples, the only thing you need to put on your breast is your baby—properly latched!

Of course, some nipple sensitivity is normal in the first seventy-two hours after birth as your breasts become used to frequent stimulation and sucking. This doesn't mean anything is wrong—in fact, it means everything is working well. Your nipples need to be sensitive to quickly send your brain the message that your baby needs milk. This releases oxytocin and prolactin, which ensure that your milk flows and that your breasts make new milk for the next feed.

While this early sensitivity is normal, you should not put up with nipple *pain*. Sometimes friends and even hospital staff say what you're doing "looks right," even when it doesn't feel right. If feeding is very painful, you must find somebody who can properly diagnose why your nipples are sore and give you the right information to make breastfeeding comfortable and enjoyable.

Friends may tell you painful nipples will get better by the time your baby is six weeks old, and this may keep you from seeking help. However, please do not put up with this unnecessary pain. Give the remedies in this chapter a try and also seek help from a La Leche League International (LLLI) counselor and/or an International Board Certified Lactation Consultant (IBCLC). Pinched, cracked, and bleeding nipples are abnormal and need emergency first aid.

When new mothers say they have painful nipples, this can mean a range of sensations. Their nipples may be:
- tender, as they sometimes feel after active foreplay
- painful like a blister
- bruised or pinched by every suck, followed by a stinging sensation after a feed
- excruciatingly painful throughout the whole feed
- deeply aching from a localized spot in the breast
- stinging and stabbing during a feed, followed by an intense burning afterward

As you can see, sore nipples involve many different levels of pain. It's really important to identify the type of pain and its cause in order to take the appropriate steps to ease it. Whenever your nipples are painful during a feed, close your eyes and imagine what's happening to your breast in your baby's mouth. How would you describe what you're feeling? Is it a tugging feeling? Does it feel as if she's pinching the tip of your nipple with her tongue? Or can you feel her tongue working along the whole length of your nipple? Slide your finger quickly into the side of your baby's mouth and push down on her bottom gum to break the suction. Look at your nipple and see if it's round or squashed. If it's pinched, the pain was telling you that she wasn't latched properly. Contact a lactation consultant and explain how your nipple felt while the baby was sucking and how your nipple looked when you took her off your breast. It's important to describe this information accurately so the consultant can diagnose what's happening in your baby's mouth and tell you how to overcome the problem.

As you'll learn in the following sections, a number of problems cause nipple pain, and you can do a number of things to solve them.

Positioning Problems

The main cause of nipple pain is holding your baby in a position that makes it difficult for her to latch easily and suck and swallow without squashing your nipple. As your milk flow becomes very fast three or four days after your baby is born, she'll almost gulp every mouthful. If her chin isn't pressing into your breast, the milk will squirt against the back of her throat, and she'll become frightened and want to stop the flow. She'll do this by squashing your nipple against the roof of her mouth, and your nipple will feel pinched at each suck.

To prevent your baby from squashing your nipple, you need to position her body firmly against yours—actually drape her against your body so her chin touches your breast. Her nose should be about a finger-width away from your breast. If her nose is pressed into your breast, put your hand between her shoulder blades to help her tilt her head back. With her chin raised and head tilted, she'll bring her tongue forward and open her throat to swallow the milk in quick mouthfuls. She'll then be able to cope with a fast flow of milk without needing to squash your nipple.

To understand why this positioning is important, try this exercise:

1. Pour a glass of water. Take a mouthful, put your chin on your chest, and swallow. The tip of your tongue will go behind your bottom gum and the rest of your tongue will push against the roof of your mouth as you tighten your throat and swallow.
2. Now take another mouthful and lift your chin to the usual drinking angle. Your tongue will go over your bottom gum so you can swallow easily. Also, your throat won't tighten as it did when your chin was on your chest.
3. If you want to gulp the water quickly, you'll need to raise your chin even higher than the usual angle, push your chin forward, and bring your tongue over your bottom gum. This will open your throat so you can swallow the water in quick gulps before you need to take a breath.

Remember that if your baby's nose is touching your breast and her chin isn't, she isn't properly positioned. You'll also know she's not latched properly if her chin is very red from rubbing up and down against your breast and if she has blisters on her top lip from turning it in to hold your breast in her mouth.

> Daniel is now two months old and doing really well. He's a very settled baby, and we're finding breastfeeding easy now. My nipples healed up, Daniel's chin lost its raw appearance, and his blistered lips returned to normal almost as soon as we used the new positioning.
>
> —Dianne

> I'm happy to report that the crack is actually *healing*—something I didn't think would really happen because feeding Alexander meant stretching, pulling, twisting, and everything else of Mom's poor nipples. Painful breastfeeding was the only thing marring the joy of Alexander's presence in our life. Now I'm so positive about it, and I really look forward to this special time together.
>
> —Eve

First-Aid Positioning for Painful Nipples

As you learned in Chapter 2 (see pages 15–20), there are many ways to position and latch your baby. When you have sore nipples due to improper positioning or any other reason, try this first-aid positioning "recipe." You'll recognize it as the cross cradle hold. Following these steps carefully will help your baby properly position and latch, and it'll provide much-needed relief for your painful nipples. Once your nipples have healed and your baby is better at latching, you can try other positioning recipes again. If you have trouble with the steps, see your lactation consultant or your local LLLI counselor for help.

1. Find a comfortable chair.
2. Start by feeding on your left breast. Lay your baby comfortably on her side, wrapping her body around your body tummy to tummy with your right arm along her back.
3. Support your baby's weight along your arm with your hand across her shoulders. Put your thumb over one shoulder and your fingers over the other so you don't hold her head. This allows your baby to tilt her head back.
4. Hold your baby very close with her nose pointing at your nipple. You need to position her so her chin is lifted and gently pushed into your breast. Her feeding reflexes and responses kick in once her chin touches your breast. She'll smell your milk and lift her mouth, which is in exactly the right place to latch.
5. Cup your left hand under your breast. Imagine your breast is a clock with twelve o'clock at the top and six o'clock at the bottom. Place your thumb on the outside edge of your areola at the three o'clock position, and your fingers on the inside edge of your breast (near your breastbone) at the nine o'clock position. Shape your areola, squeezing your breast so it's parallel to your baby's lips.
6. Point your nipple to her nose.
7. Rub the underside of your areola on your baby's bottom lip, keeping the nipple above her top lip. As her mouth rubs across your areola, the nipple may become erect and the skin of the areola may crinkle and tighten. Wait until this tightness passes and the nipple and areola soften before continuing.

8. Watch for:
   - her mouth to open wide,
   - her tongue to come forward over her bottom gum, and
   - her bottom lip to turn down on your breast.

   At this point, bring your baby quickly toward you, with your wrist flat against her shoulder blades.

9. Keep your breast shaped while she takes eight to ten sucks. Flip out her top lip with your thumb if it's not already turned out. Move your hand away to put it under her body to cradle her.

10. Relax. If you like, support your baby on a pillow now that she's latched. Using a pillow before latching often creates problems with both positioning and latching.

11. Now try on your right breast. Repeat the same steps, only this time using your left arm around her back and your right hand to shape your breast. This time, your thumb will be at nine o'clock and your fingers at three 'clock.

Daniel and I are eagerly learning our new latching techniques. He's more settled at the right breast, and I'm not experiencing pain of any significance. Thank God! In the face of persistent difficulties, breastfeeding can be quite demoralizing, but you can't sit on your hands—you have to apply new learning. It's a deep pleasure to feed my beautiful boy, as it's one of the best legacies I can give him. Thanks for your help at a very anxious time.

—Ruth

Yes, as you've no doubt guessed, the absence of telephone calls does mean Daniel is like the kitten who got the cream and I'm a very happy mom who feels like a conqueror! The last few weeks of our happy liaison have been wonderful. I'm enjoying feeding him, and we're developing a lovely synchrony. As we start a feed he gets really excited—his legs squirm around and he puts his hands on my breast to help himself latch.

—Ruth (two months later)

We're doing fine with breastfeeding now. The painful feeding improved within a few days of your suggestion to change the positioning and latching. We had a few ups and downs with how I held him over the next couple of weeks, but finally we got it worked out. Thank goodness—life is much easier now! No one ever told me establishing breast-feeding could be more difficult than childbirth!

—Kerry

Nose Blockage

After birth, some babies have mucus suctioned from their noses and throats. Suction irritates the lining of the nose and throat, which reacts by producing extra mucus. If this happened to your baby, her nose may be plugged, and she may not be able to suck properly during feeding. If you've ever had a stuffy nose, you know how hard it can be to eat and breathe at the same time. When your baby has a stuffy nose, she'll get frightened because she can't breathe when her mouth is full of your breast. She'll push your breast out of her mouth a bit so she can breathe through her mouth. This means she'll squash your nipple painfully up against her hard palate (see page 92). This also means your baby won't drink enough milk to be satisfied because she doesn't have enough of the breast in her mouth. She'll then be very unsettled and will want to feed very often.

If your baby is latching poorly because of a stuffy nose, it's expressed breastmilk to the rescue! Expressed breastmilk is not just yummy and very good for babies to drink, it's also helpful in overcoming problems such as blocked noses and sticky eyes (a condition in which the tear duct is blocked, causing discharge). Express about twenty drops of your milk and collect them in a carefully cleaned eyedropper or syringe. Encourage your baby to suck on your clean, short-nailed little finger (nail-side down toward her tongue). While she sucks, gently place a few drops of milk into each nostril—she'll simply swallow the milk as it runs down the back of her throat. If she coughs, stop. After she swallows the milk, twirl the corner of a tissue so it's firm enough to put into her nose to remove the mucus. Usually, you'll need to do this only once, and your baby will then breathe well and feed without hurting your nipples.

Overactive Gag Reflex and Thumb or Fist Sucking

When babies are born, their bottom gums are a little behind their top gums. For your baby to milk your breast well and not hurt your nipple, the tip of your nipple needs to be at the junction of her hard and soft palates. To learn where this is, feel the roof of your mouth (your palate) by running your finger or tongue along it. It feels hard until you come to a ridge quite a way back, and it then inclines and feels softer. Your breast is in the right position when the tip of your nipple is at this junction in your baby's mouth. This position allows your baby to build up suction in her mouth.[2] Her tongue will be flat, and she'll milk your breast with a rhythmic rolling motion from the front to the back of her tongue. But if your baby has an overactive gag reflex or is a thumb or fist sucker, she won't keep

your nipple at that junction, which means she'll try to milk your nipple instead of your breast. This not only causes you pain but also keeps her from getting enough to drink, which means she'll constantly cry and want to feed.

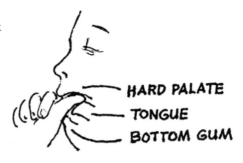

The gag reflex is very important to babies because it closes their throats and causes their tongues to push out anything unwanted in their mouths. If your baby had mucus sucked out of her nose and mouth at birth, she may hate having anything, including your breast, in her mouth. This will trigger the overactive gag reflex. Even if you latch her properly, she'll get frightened, gag, and push your breast to a more comfortable spot for her—which will be a very uncomfortable spot for you.

Fist and thumb suckers often create the same problems with breastfeeding. If your baby sucked her fist during an ultrasound or she put her thumb into her mouth as soon as she was born, I'm sure you thought it was really cute. This well-ingrained habit often starts at about eighteen weeks into pregnancy, so by full-term, your baby may have been sucking her fist or thumb for over twenty weeks. Sucking a thumb or fist is different from sucking a breast, so during a feed, she'll push your breast out of her mouth to suck the way she's learned. This means she'll suck your nipple and not your breast. To help you understand the way she sucks, try the following:

- Put your thumb into your mouth and suck on it. You'll find that you put it only part of the way along your hard palate and push against it with your tongue. The back of your tongue rubs against your hard and soft palate.
- Make a fist and suck on the side of your first finger or thumb. The tip of your tongue won't hold your flesh in your mouth but will push it in and out.

If your baby has an overactive gag reflex or sucks her thumb or fist, she not only sucks in a different way than she needs to, but she probably also doesn't open her mouth wide enough. You or your partner can use the following massage technique to help her overcome her sensitive gag reflex, teach her to use her feeding responses correctly, and open her mouth wide. Continue to do this exercise for no longer than thirty seconds before each feed and when she's happily awake until your nipples are no longer painful.

1. Wash your hands.
2. Sit on a comfortable chair with your feet on a footstool so your knees make a lap.
3. Put your baby facing you on a pillow on your lap.
4. Firmly stroke from her cheekbone to the corner of her mouth to encourage her rooting reflex. To avoid confusing her, stroke only one side of her face each time. She'll turn her head side to side and search with her mouth.
5. Using a finger wet with expressed breastmilk, firmly massage her bottom lip and chin to simulate your breast rubbing on them.
6. When she opens her mouth, rub the tip of her tongue to encourage her to poke it out. (This is called the extrusion reflex.) The tip of the tongue is very sensitive, and with a lot of massage, she'll start to poke it out over her bottom gum and lip. Because babies can mimic from birth, poke out your tongue while doing this massage to show her what she needs to do.
7. If her gums, jaw, and hands are tight, massage the inside of her lips with a wet finger. This will release oxytocin to relax her.
8. Once she brings her tongue forward, you can pop your clean, short-nailed little finger into her mouth, nail-side down toward her tongue.

Slowly move your finger back along her hard palate until you almost reach the soft palate. It's important not to press down on her tongue, as this will make her gag.

9. If this exercise makes her gag, slow down and start again. Otherwise, she won't want anything in her mouth. If she does gag, take note of how far your finger was in her mouth when it happened. Start again and move your finger up to the spot where she gagged. Let her suck contentedly for a while, then gradually start the massage again, slowly moving your finger back to where the hard and soft palate meet. This is where the tip of your nipple needs to be for pain-free feeding.

10. If your baby is happy to keep sucking, let her do so. This will get her used to having something this far in her mouth, and she'll learn to keep her tongue flat in order to suck. If you like, you can reward your baby by gently dropping some breastmilk from a syringe or eyedropper down the side of your finger so she swallows about every two seconds and learns a good suck-swallow-breathe sequence.

Nipple Thrush

If you're prone to thrush (candidiasis or yeast infection), you may acquire this very painful fungal condition in the breast after you've taken antibiotics. (Antibiotics kill good bacteria as well as bad, and in the absence of good bacteria, yeast tends to flourish.) Young babies also often have thrush in their mouths, which can appear as white patches on the inside of their cheeks, on their gums, and on their tongues. If this is the case with you or your baby, you'll need to treat your nipples as well as her mouth because thrush is easily transmitted.

Thrush causes a hot, searing pain throughout the feed that may also radiate deep into the breast, and this burning continues after feeding. You may suspect you have thrush if:

- Your nipples suddenly become painful when you haven't had any other nipple pain since you began breastfeeding.
- Your nipples are painful right through the feed and even worse when the feed has finished.
- Your nipples are a pink-orange color and very dry.

If you and your baby have thrush, it's important to get treatment right away because this pain won't just go away. If you have some plain yogurt in the fridge, put a little on your nipples and cover them with soft pads. This will be soothing first aid until you can talk to your caregiver or lactation consultant, who'll most likely recommend an over-the-counter antifungal ointment containing miconazole. You should use it on your nipples and in your baby's mouth as directed at least four times every twenty-four hours. You can get the ointment as a gel or cream. For your baby, use the gel form. Respected Australian lactation consultant Bridget Ingle says it works better if you first wipe your baby's tongue with a clean, wet face cloth before applying the gel in your baby's mouth. If the gel irritates your nipples, change to a cream for your own use. (Continue using the gel for your baby.) Apply only a very small amount, and rub it well into your nipples. Ingle also suggests using baking soda (sodium bicarbonate) nipple rinses. Four times a day, put one teaspoon of baking soda in a cup of water and splash it on your nipples. Splash warm water over them to rinse them before the next feed.

If you have thrush, try to lower the level of yeast (candida) in your body by adding yogurt to your diet, eating foods with less sugar and yeast, and taking acidophilus capsules. To prevent reinfection, carefully scrub your nails and wash your hands after changing and feeding your baby. Wash your underclothes and bras daily, and if possible, dry them in sunlight.

> If you think you have thrush from taking an antibiotic, talk to your caregiver. It may be caused by an incorrect antibiotic, or you may in fact have a bacterial infection such as staph (staphylococcus aureus) instead of thrush. See pages 104–105 for more details.

Milk under the Skin

Sometimes skin grows over a nipple pore, causing milk to back up behind the skin and thicken. Researchers suggest this overgrowth of tissue is due to the high levels of epidermal growth factor (EGF) in breastmilk. Milk under the skin develops as a painful white spot on your nipple about the size of a pinhead, though sometimes larger. Some mothers have general breast tenderness but no nipple pain, while others have mild to severe burning pain in their nipples and the breast during and immediately after feeding.[3]

Sometimes these spots open during a feed, and your baby will clear the thickened milk. If this doesn't happen, you'll need to break the skin and open the nipple pore with a sterile needle to let the milk flow. If you don't wish to do this yourself, ask your partner to help or see your caregiver or lactation consultant. These spots often become more prominent and easier to treat if your baby feeds for a couple of minutes before you attempt to break the skin. Expressing or continuing the feed after you break the skin ensures that the thickened milk is removed.

Vasospasm of the Nipple

Vasospasm of the nipple, first recognized by Laureen and Carolyn Lawlor-Smith, is a variant of Raynaud's disease, a condition in which cold or stress causes the arteries in one's extremities (usually fingers or toes) to constrict.[4] This makes the skin go numb and turn white then blue, and then become very painful and red as circulation returns. If you have vasospasm in your nipples, you'll experience intermittent pain and changes in nipple color. You'll feel numbness, tingling, and then burning pain during feeding. After the feed, your nipples will be white or in severe cases will turn blue. As your circulation returns, you'll feel an intense burning, and your nipples will become red before returning to their usual color.

If this happens to you, try the following tips:

- Keep your whole body warm and wear extra-warm underclothes to keep your breasts warm. Make some lambskin nipple pads to wear.
- Breastfeed in a warm room.
- Hold a warm (not hot) pack against your breasts at the end of each feed.
- Talk to your caregiver about a six-week course of fish oil or evening primrose oil. Laureen Lawlor-Smith reports that these supplements can help if taken for six weeks, but shorter courses have not been shown to be helpful.
- Quit smoking—even two cigarettes a day can affect your circulation. Caffeine and decongestants also have this effect.
- Seek medical advice from your caregiver, because medication (containing nifedipine) may be helpful.

Short-Term Expressing for Painful Nipples

Many mothers with sore nipples dread feeding their babies at the breast because they're afraid of more pain. In many cases, though, the best remedy for painful nipples is to put your baby on your breast—properly. But if you've tried many ways to overcome your nipple pain and nothing has worked, you may decide to rest your nipples for a day or two. Expressing and feeding the milk to your baby can help because a pump (or hand-expressing) uses a perfect "latch" that won't hurt your nipples. After a few days, you can put your baby back on the breast. In the meantime, here are a few ways you can feed your baby while you give your nipples a rest.

Cup- or Spoon-Feeding

Babies can cup-feed from birth. To do this, wrap your baby so she can't knock the cup, and sit her in a semi-upright position in the crook of your arm. Put a small quantity of your milk into a small, clean cup. Rest the cup on your baby's bottom lip and slowly tip it so some drops of milk run into her mouth. She'll quickly learn to bring her tongue forward and lap the milk from the lip of the cup as you slowly tilt it. Continue to put small amounts of milk into the cup and feed her until she's full. Spoon-feeding is another option, and it's done in much the same way as with a cup. The slow tilting of the spoon helps your baby to lap and cope easily with the flow.

Talk to your lactation consultant or your baby's caregiver to learn how much your baby needs at each feeding. You can also work it out by multiplying her weight by two and a half ounces and dividing that amount by the number of feeds in twenty-four hours. For example, if your baby weighs seven pounds (7 x 2.5 = 17.5 ounces) and you normally feed eight times a day (17.5 ounces ÷ 8 feeds), you'll need about two ounces of milk per feed.

Bottle-Feeding

When sucking on bottles, babies use their tongues, cheeks, and jaws quite differently than when they suck on breasts. When breastfeeding, your baby's tongue is flat, and she brings it forward over her bottom gum. She milks the breast with rhythmic waves from the front to the back of her tongue. Her jaws work with a slow opening-and-closing movement. When feeding from a bottle, a baby puts the tip of her tongue behind her bottom gum and pushes the back of her tongue against the roof of her mouth to slow the flow from the bottle nipple. This is exactly what your baby's tongue does when it painfully pinches your nipples at each suck. If you feed your baby from a bottle when giving your nipples a rest, it'll only encourage her to continue believing this is the way to suck.

However, if you decide bottle-feeding your expressed milk is the most practical thing to do until your nipples heal, buy a long latex nipple (if available). Start the feed with her head tilted back, and massage her lips with the bottle nipple or your finger to encourage her to open her mouth wide. As often as possible, feed her against your bare breast so returning to the breast will be a natural progression. You may think this hiatus will be a good time for your partner to feed the baby, but that can come later, when you return to work or activities outside the home and you and your baby are both breastfeeding pros.

Going Back to the Breast

When your nipples feel more comfortable and you put your baby back on the breast, you can judge how much better she's latching by rating the pain on a one (least painful) to ten (most painful) scale. The lower the number, the better the latch. Don't leave her on the breast if your pain level is above five, as this usually means she's pinching the tip of your nipple. With good advice and assistance from your lactation consultant, within one or two feeds your score should be down to two or three. Of course, your target is a zero rating with no pain at all, but sometimes the bruising and tenderness will take a few feeds to disappear completely.

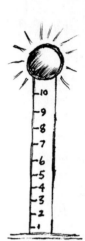

I always imagined I would breastfeed, but I had no idea what a battle it would be. The crack on the right side opened up all the time and just wouldn't heal. I dreaded putting James on that side, which made me realize perhaps I wasn't pushing him on far enough. So I gave it a better try, and things improved a little. I had been feeding sitting up in bed, not wanting to risk incorrect positioning, but I was just too tired two nights ago, so I lay down and carefully put him on. Magic! I suppose his tongue was rubbing in the right place, and the crack didn't open. About four feeds later, my nipple was looking great! It healed almost overnight, and both nipples are now nice and rosy pink. The pain is down to a two. We didn't quite make it to zero by the time James was two weeks old, as I had hoped. But I'm predicting—and being very generous—that we'll be down to zero pain and perfect feeding on both sides when he's one month old. When you're having problems, the bottle starts looking good, but I would have been truly disappointed to give up breastfeeding.

—Jenny

Painful Breasts

As with painful nipples, you may have painful breasts for a number of reasons while breastfeeding. Whatever the reason, the most important thing to do is to continue draining your breasts completely at feeds and get lots of rest and support. Here are some common causes of—and solutions for—painful breasts. As you'll see, one problem can cascade into the next unless you take proper steps to treat your condition.

Blocked Duct

The most common cause of painful breasts is not properly draining your breasts. Fat globules clump together to cause a blockage in your duct, and milk builds up behind it, creating a painful lump and inflammation in the breast. This is different than when you have a blocked nipple pore and milk under the skin (see pages 95–96).

When you have a blocked duct, your milk often tastes salty. This sets up a vicious cycle in which your baby doesn't feed well on that breast for a day or two, your breast doesn't drain, and your milk continues to get saltier. As the poor feeding continues, you'll feel as if you're getting the flu—you'll have a headache, general body aches, shivers, and tiredness. You may have a small lump and a pink area on your breast.

The best "medicine" is to rest, feed your baby, and eat and drink well, so you'll need someone to help you for a day or two. Also, make an appointment with your caregiver, but in the meantime, try some first aid with the following tips:

- Eat freshly crushed garlic either mixed with food or on toast. Research has shown that babies like garlic-flavored milk.[5] The garlic will cover the salty taste, and your baby will probably drain your breast better. Garlic is also considered to be a natural antibacterial agent and may prevent the inflammation from becoming an infection (mastitis).
- Place a warm pack (wrapped in a cloth so you don't burn yourself) over the sore spot. This will bring a good blood supply to the spot and increase your oxytocin level, which will help extra milk unblock the duct as you feed.

- Take a mild over-the-counter anti-inflammatory tablet such as ibuprofen to relieve the pain, and go to bed.

At the next feed, try these tips:

- Feed your baby from the sore side with her chin pointing to the sore spot.
- Lie down to feed, leaning on your elbow above your baby so your breast falls forward.
- Massage the sore spot from behind and down toward your nipple as she feeds.
- Feed from the other breast or express milk from it to keep it comfortable and healthy.
- When your breast has drained, sleep until the next feed.
- If it's too painful to feed your baby, use a breast pump, leaning forward while you express so the breast falls forward and drains better. Or have your partner latch on and drink the milk until the breast is drained and feels soft and comfortable.

Thanks so much for your advice about breast drainage! After trying all the usual things to get rid of the lumps and feeling very anxious about developing mastitis, it was a great relief to discover that when all else fails, I can clear the lumps at home with the help of a happily obliging husband! Now if I get a lump, my husband is quick to help, and the lumps disappear. The other thing I remember you saying is "A rest a day keeps the lumps away"...and it does!

—Melinda

If your breast looks and feels better after these tips, you can probably cancel your appointment and continue with the first-aid care. However, if your breast is now quite red, more swollen, and more painful, then you must visit your caregiver because you likely have mastitis. You'll feel very sick and will probably need somebody to help you with your baby and drive you to your appointment.

Mastitis

Blocked ducts and mastitis (a bacterial infection of the breast) are very common in our society, where a new mother typically has little family support and may become tired and stressed no matter how loving, helpful, and supportive her partner is. Being run-down is one of the major causes of mastitis.

The most likely treatment for mastitis will be:

- Pain-relief medication—some caregivers now routinely prescribe anti-inflammatory medication, which relieves pain and reduces the inflammation of your breast.
- Antibiotic therapy with penicillinase-resistant penicillin (used for penicillin-resistant staphylococcus aureus) for seven to ten days.
- Ultrasound treatment by your caregiver or a physiotherapist to help the milk flow. The swelling will increase if you don't feed your baby or drain your breast with a good pump right after the treatment.
- Continuation of the first-aid care suggested for a blocked duct (see pages 100–101).

Things to Do

While on antibiotics (which kill good bacteria along with the bad), eat yogurt that contains acidophilus and bifidobacterium or take acidophilus powder to replace your body's good bacteria. This can help prevent yeast infection and digestive troubles. Also, if you're using oral contraception, remember that antibiotics may reduce its effectiveness, so use a backup barrier method as well.

When your treatment is complete, take the following precautions to prevent another case of mastitis:

- For the first six weeks after birth, try not to get involved in too many things outside your home. Historically, women of the family cared for new mothers for six weeks.
- Stay seated until you finish each feed. Plan how to cope with distractions, including the telephone, doorbell, and your other children.
- Break up long journeys. If you travel a long way to visit grandparents or friends, your baby may sleep while your breasts fill, and your seat

belt will pull tighter and tighter over them. Stop your journey and wake your baby for a feed.

- Wear clothes that don't constrict your breasts. You create pressure on your breast and stop milk from draining when you wear strapless dresses, wear bras with lots of seams, and pull tight clothing up into your armpits while feeding.

- Take a nap. Leave the housework and cooking to your partner or another support person, and sleep for an hour or lie down to feed your baby so you're completely relaxed.

- Care for your body. Although your breasts make milk even if you don't eat properly, your body—like any other machine—needs fuel to keep going. Make a point of eating breakfast, as this will give you energy to do the morning chores. Lunch is also important. Make this the main meal of the day so you'll have lots of energy for the evening, when your baby will want to spend a lot of time with you. Try to have supper early, even if that means eating alone before your partner gets home from work. Your energy level will be too low if you wait until seven or eight o'clock.

- Accept help when it's offered. This is probably the most difficult thing to do because women like to be independent and are likely to say, "No, thank you. I'll be fine." Your new line should be, "Yes, please. I would love you to do that!"

After a bout of mastitis, I've finally found the inner resources to start some decent lifestyle and wellness activities, such as eating sensibly, doing aerobics, and so on. It's amazing how much energy you have when you're well! It's been really scary living with persistent tiredness and lack of energy from not eating properly or exercising.

—Annette

Breast Abscess

A breast abscess can occur if the antibiotic you've been taking for mastitis is ineffective against the bacteria or if you have continued with daily ultrasound treatments when your blocked duct has not cleared. Your breast becomes very red and extremely painful, and you'll need to be admitted to the hospital for intravenous antibiotics, needle drainage of the abscess, or even surgery to drain the abscess.

If you need to have surgery, it's important to ask the surgeon if it's possible for the incision to be made over the abscess site but far enough from your areola so you can continue to breastfeed. After the operation, there's no reason why you can't breastfeed your baby at her next feed. It won't be unbearably painful because you'll have good pain relief—most hospital pharmacies now have the latest information on medications that are safe for breastfeeding—particularly from Thomas Hale's *Medications and Mothers' Milk* (see pages 111–112).[6] Feeding will in fact make your breast feel better very quickly because it will remove milk and reduce pressure on the abscess spot. If your baby can't be with you, you'll need to express or pump.

When you feed, milk will come out of your breast where the cut was made as well as through your nipple. This leakage will probably continue for a few weeks while the cut gradually heals. The leak bathes the new tissue in milk, which contains epidermal growth factor and other factors that prevent infections and help new cells grow quickly.

Thrush in the Breast...Or Is It a Bacterial Infection?

You can get thrush (a yeast infection) in your nipple (see pages 94–95) as well as your breast. If you're prone to thrush, you may get it in your breast after taking antibiotics. Thrush in the breast causes a hot, searing pain deep in the breast during feeds, and the burning feeling continues after the feed.

If you suspect thrush caused by antibiotics, see your caregiver. It's important to investigate your breast pain, as it may not be due to too many antibiotics but instead incorrect antibiotics—or possibly it's not thrush but a bacterial infection such as staph (staphylococcus aureus).

As with nipple thrush, it may be helpful to lower the level of yeast (candida) in your body by adding yogurt to your diet, eating foods with less sugar and yeast, and taking acidophilus capsules. You may also find it helpful to rub nystatin ointment onto the painful parts of your breasts as well as onto your areola and nipples three or four times a day after feeding. Gently and carefully wash your nipples and areola before feeds to remove the ointment.

I feel I've had every problem in the book as far as breastfeeding is concerned. It all started with a slightly inverted right nipple. This wasn't a big problem, but Caitlan had a bit of trouble latching on. Eventually when the milk came in, the nipple popped out by itself. As Caitlan's suck grew stronger, I started to have severe pains when she first latched on. (People said it was because I have a very fair complexion, but that's an old wives' tale.) This led to cracked nipples, which caused more pain and made my right nipple bleed. Caitlan swallowed the blood, and she vomited. I started crying—the whole thing was a fiasco!

The next thing I knew, I was in the hospital with a uterine infection. I also had blocked ducts and engorgement in the troublesome right breast. I was so nervous in the emergency room, I leaked all over my hospital gown. It was so saturated, you could have wrung it out!

I was in the hospital for four days, and I had to pump my breasts most of the time because I wasn't allowed to keep the baby with me. My husband could bring her in only once or twice a day. I pumped four ounces every three to four hours. Everyone was amazed at how much milk I had, and they called me "K's Dairy." Some nurses said I had extra milk because I'm an Aussie! The four days of expressing in the hospital gave my nipples a chance to heal.

When I went home, the pain during feeding seemed to go away, but then I suddenly had a different pain—a burning from the back of my breasts. All the antibiotics I had had in the hospital had caused thrush. Both Caitlan and I had to be treated for it. Then I started having more problems with her pinching my nipples, so my La Leche League leader helped me learn to position her.

I had just conquered these problems when I got my first period and my milk suddenly decreased. After all I'd been through, I was so afraid my milk had dried up and I'd have to give up breastfeeding! I took all the advice from my lactation consultant (feed more often, rest, drink fluids, massage the breast, and so on), and now I seem to have enough to satisfy Caitlan's increasing hunger.

It was disappointing to find out that breastfeeding is not as "natural" and instinctive as I had first believed. I'm glad I persevered, though. It was worth the effort because now I feel warm and wonderful when I feed Caitlan. Thank heavens I'm so stubborn and have such a loving mother to support me, or I would have never managed to get through it!

—Kathy

Ingestion and Digestion Problems

Not all breastfeeding problems involve nipple or breast pain. Some problems stem from how babies ingest and digest breastmilk, as you'll see here.

Rapid Milk Flow

"Wow, Mom…it's great milk, but can you slow it down?" For some babies, the arrival of milk in large quantities can be a bit scary. Even for babies who've learned a good suck-swallow-breathe sequence, sometimes milk flow can be so fast that they push their tongues up against their hard palates to stop the flow (see page 92). This is very painful for the mothers, and it's no fun for babies, either.

If your baby seems to have trouble keeping up with your milk flow, try these tips to help her cope with it:

- Watch her sucking pattern. If she starts to make a crowing noise or coughs and sputters early in the feed, detach her by quickly putting your finger in the side of her mouth. Have a cloth close by to catch the spray of milk as she detaches from your breast. When the spray stops, let her latch again, or help her if necessary, making sure you have her positioned so her head tilts well back, her chin points into your breast, and her nose is well away from your breast. Let her latch and detach a few times until the flow of milk slows. Even in this exaggerated position, your baby may still cough and sputter.

- Hold her in a semi-upright sitting position, with her legs astride your thighs and your hand behind her shoulders so her chin is well into your breast and her nose is away from it. She may be able to manage the flow more easily in this position than when she's lying down.

- Try lying down on your back with your baby on top of you. If it's hard to latch your baby this way, try sitting up to latch, then sliding down onto your back. After five minutes, sit up and make sure your baby remains well latched for the rest of the feed.

- Express until the first milk ejection has subsided. Your baby may cope better with the less forceful ejections that follow.

Nipple Shields

Some babies can't swallow quickly enough even when their mothers use the milk-flow management strategies described on page 106. If this is the case with your baby, try using a nipple shield. This is a silicone shield shaped like an areola and nipple, and some kinds have one or two sides cut away so the baby can feel your bare breast instead of silicone against her chin. You place the shield over your areola and nipple. The shield has only three holes in its tip, which will slow the flow of milk. To attach it correctly, imagine putting on a sock: turn it halfway inside out, stretch it open, and roll it onto your nipple, flattening the edges against your areola. As you roll it on, it will draw your nipple into the shield and make a seal. If you don't use this method, it'll slide around the breast because of the fast jets of milk behind it.

Nipple shields can be a boon if your milk flow is too fast, but they can be dangerous if you use them when you have a low supply of milk or when your baby has trouble getting enough milk at each feed. If you're using a nipple shield and it has lowered your milk supply, then your baby may lie at your breast and suck for hours without getting enough milk.

> I just wanted to let you know that at twelve months, I'm still breastfeeding my son, Julian, with a nipple shield! Julian and I have both benefited from breastfeeding in so many ways. I want to let you know that I noticed how nipple shields change with repeated use and particularly with sterilization. It was okay for Julian, but from my side of the silicon I could feel his suckling much better on thinner, newer shields. I think this may be important for newer babies with ongoing feeding problems.
>
> —Melinda

On rare occasions, there's no way to slow fast-flowing milk, and some mothers go on to bottle-feed their expressed milk at all feeds. In order to maintain your milk supply, follow the advice on pages 55–58 about frequency of expression. Even if you can't feed at the breast, you'll still want to make feeding time special. You should always be the person to bottle-feed during the first month or two so your baby can enjoy your face, your smell, your voice, and the feel of your soft skin during this important bonding time.

You need to hold your baby as close as possible in the crook of your arm with her face no more than eight inches from yours so she can see you easily. Breastfeeding is often seen just as a way to give babies nutrition, when in fact it's also a way to nurture babies through sensory input and loving contact. For many years, research has shown that body contact from a constant caregiver is essential to the normal development of babies.[7] This special contact is also good for mothers. You may feel as if you're missing out on the joy of breastfeeding if all you can do is express and hand the baby and the bottle to someone else. Having this special bond at feeding time for the first month or so will help you have a more positive experience.

> I'm writing to thank you for all your help in the first weeks after Natalie was born. Because of your commitment, I regard myself as a success, and I'm determined to continue expressing. It seems like only yesterday when I said I wanted to express for at least three months if possible. Now, five and a half months have flown by, and I'm still managing. With each and every bottle I express, I feel a sense of satisfaction. I feel sorry for those mothers who've had breastfeeding trouble—and I realize so many out there are unaware of the different things you can do to make sure babies get their mothers' precious milk.
>
> —Deborah

Lactose Intolerance

Nonhuman mammals and most of the world's population do not drink milk after weaning. In humans, lactase—the enzyme that breaks down lactose (the main sugar in milk)—declines between three and five years of age, and people can develop an intolerance to milk at that time. Lactose intolerance is normal in most of the world's children and adults.

Some parents falsely assume that because they're lactose intolerant, their babies will be, too. Actually, it's very rare for babies to inherit an inability to digest lactose. You'll remember from Chapter 1 (see page 7) that lactose is necessary for brain growth. However, lactose intolerance can become a temporary problem if you or your baby has been treated with antibiotics or she has had diarrhea. Instead of the normal watery, mustard-colored stool at every feed, your baby will have frothy gray-green stool. She'll also feed very frequently, not gain weight, and have a very nasty diaper rash.

If your baby is diagnosed with lactose intolerance, this isn't time to wean. If your baby's caregiver suggests lactose-free formula for this temporary problem, continue breastfeeding but give your baby the formula once a day at the feed before her longest sleep. For a more severe case, use the lactose-free formula at alternate feeds—give her breastmilk at one feed and formula at the next. In a very severe case, you may need to give your baby lactose-free formula at all feeds for some weeks so her bowel can rest. If you express your milk and freeze it during this time, you can gradually reintroduce breastmilk later.

Lactose Overload

While lactose intolerance is rare in babies, lactose overload may happen if you have a large milk supply and you breastfeed only for short times on each breast at each feed. As you'll remember in Chapter 5 (see pages 75–76), some babies need to swap breasts frequently when they have weight-gain problems. But if you've been feeding for short periods from each breast and your baby hasn't had a weight-gain problem, this may cause lactose overload. This makes your baby want to feed very often, spit up after feeds, pass lots of gas, constantly suck her fist, and have "explosive" mustard-colored stools and very heavy wet diapers.

In 1984, I researched this problem and found that when babies with lactose overload drank from only one breast at each feed, they became more settled, and normal eliminating patterns returned. This is because a baby receives creamy hind milk when she drains a breast, and that milk goes through her gut much more slowly than lots of low-fat fore milk. Some mothers used this method for a couple of days, some for a couple of weeks, some for a couple of months, and some for a couple of years. They often went back to using both breasts at each feed when the diapers were less wet and their babies stopped gaining weight.

> One of the most difficult things has been whether to use
> one or both breasts at each feed. When Jordan had very
> squirty stool, you suggested I use just one breast at each feed
> so he would get all the milk out of that breast. It worked.
> After a couple of weeks, he wanted more than just one breast
> at a feed, but he never really made the second one as soft
> as the first. I worried about whether he was still getting enough
> creamy milk, but he didn't get the squirty problem again, so I
> guess nature worked it all out. The hardest part of motherhood
> has been stopping myself from analyzing everything—just as I
> spent the past fifteen years analyzing everything at work!
>
> —Sarah

"Colic," Food Intolerance, and Food Allergies

Too much lactose can give babies a lot of gas in their bowels. This in turn
causes "overstretching" of the bowels. Particularly in the early weeks of life,
some babies find it difficult to cope with this swelling, so they cry because
of their discomfort. Other babies may be affected by an intolerance or
allergy to a food in their mothers' diet—for example, cow milk.

Sometimes people identify these situations as "colic," though we don't
really know what causes colic or if such a condition even exists. Colic has
become a loose term to describe the condition of any baby that cries a lot,
but true colic, whatever its cause may be, is diagnosed by the type of crying.[8]
A baby with true colic will:

- Cry for three hours a day for more than three days in a week.
- Cry for a few minutes, suddenly stop, and then suddenly start again
  (which is called paroxysm of crying).

Some people suggest breastfeeding mothers shouldn't eat certain foods
because they might make the babies gassy. Very little research has been
done on the subject, but some babies do improve when their mothers
remove cow milk from their diets. Regardless of whether mothers change
their diets, the crying and discomfort usually just decrease over time.
(What we do know about breastfeeding and mothers' diets is that babies
like their mothers to continue eating the foods they ate in pregnancy. The

foods you ate during pregnancy flavored your amniotic fluid, which your baby drank, so she's familiar with those tastes.)

If your baby has colic-like symptoms, it's of course important to rule out medical causes, but research has shown that medicating babies is less effective than supporting parents.[9] If your baby cries frequently, your tension can add to her distress. Having your partner or a support person take your baby so you can unwind during her crying spells can help immensely. The popular treatment of giving babies herbal teas for colic is now discouraged because they often contain chamomile, which is associated with sudden infant death syndrome (SIDS). In cultures where babies are constantly carried in an upright position, there's no word for *colic*; perhaps because these babies aren't fed and then laid down to sleep. We adults often have pain if we nap after eating, so it's plausible that babies feel the same discomfort. Carrying your baby in a sling after each feed during daylight hours might help.

Transfer of Medications and Recreational Drugs

Some medications and most recreational drugs are harmful when transferred to a baby through breastmilk. If you're using either, learn more about how it affects your breastmilk and your baby.

Medications

We've made great advances in our knowledge about the transfer of medications into breastmilk. Most medications transfer into milk, but at minimal concentration—generally 1 percent of your dose. This is often far too low to produce any effect on your breastfed baby. A medication has to pass lots of barriers to get to your baby. It has to:

- survive the acid in your stomach
- be absorbed into your blood supply
- pass from your blood supply into your milk
- survive the high acid content of your baby's stomach
- be absorbed into your baby's blood supply

If your caregiver prescribes medication while you're breastfeeding, find out as much as possible about it. Make sure your caregiver knows you're breastfeeding, and ask him or her to read about the medication in Thomas Hale's *Medications and Mothers' Milk*. This is the most up-to-date research-based book on the subject, and it states whether a medication is approved by the American Academy of Pediatrics (AAP) for use by breastfeeding mothers.

The most important thing you can do to reduce the amount of a medication your baby gets through your milk is to take it immediately after a feed. If it isn't safe to expose your baby to your medication, you may be able to express and discard your milk until your medication is completed or changed. During this time, you can feed your baby your previously expressed and stored milk, donated milk from a milk bank, or hypoallergenic formula.

Things to Do

To ensure that your baby isn't unnecessarily exposed to medications:
✔ Use menthol-steam inhalators instead of oral antihistamines or decongestants when you have a cold.
✔ Use creams instead of tablets for skin irritations.
✔ Use nasal drops instead of tablets for sinus problems.

Caffeine, Nicotine, Alcohol, and Marijuana

Caffeine, nicotine, alcohol, and marijuana (cannabis) are all drugs widely used in the twenty-first century. Caffeine from tea, coffee, colas, or chocolate may transfer to your baby if you have excessive amounts. If your normal intake is three or four caffeinated drinks or a small amount of chocolate a day, it'll probably have little effect on her. However, if your baby is very unsettled, it may be worth reducing your caffeine intake.

If you're a smoker, the most important thing you can do is quit because nicotine does transfer to your baby, as do many of the other harmful substances in cigarettes. If you're finding it difficult to stop while breast-feeding, it's preferable to smoke after a feed and not in the same room as your baby. This will reduce the amount of nicotine your baby takes in through your milk and the air. Research results show that wearing low-level nicotine patches reduces the amount of nicotine in breastmilk and may be better than continuing to smoke.[10] If you can't quit smoking and patches aren't helpful to you, then breastfeeding is still the best thing for you and your baby.

In the first three or four days after birth, alcohol enters your milk very easily, so save any celebratory champagne until the end of the first week. Occasional moderate drinking after that time has not been shown to harm babies. Your milk alcohol level is roughly the same as your blood alcohol level, so after a drink or two, your milk contains up to 0.1 percent alcohol. Certainly, heavy drinking may cause problems for your baby. Some babies don't like the taste of alcohol in breastmilk and drink less milk in the four hours after their mothers have imbibed.[11] Alcohol may also make your baby sleepy and dehydrated. If your baby seems to be reacting poorly to your alcohol use, you may need to either cut back or time your drinking more carefully. It takes two hours for your body to break down one standard drink and for your blood (and milk) alcohol level to drop to zero. So if you'd really like to have a drink, the best time to do it is immediately after a feed. Many people will tell you that an alcoholic drink—stout, in particular—will help your milk supply. Research by Julie Mennella has shown this to be incorrect.[12]

Marijuana is absorbed into fat and stays in your brain for at least a month. If you breastfeed, it'll stay in your baby's brain for even longer. If you abstained during pregnancy, then it's important to continue abstaining while breastfeeding. All addictive drugs penetrate your milk and stay in your baby's body much longer than they do in yours. There may be a legal consequence if your baby is screened for drugs and found to be positive.

An Important Message about Breastfeeding Problems

It seems you can encounter a mountain of problems during breastfeeding, and many new mothers encounter at least one. As Jenny mentioned in her letter on page 99, the bottle—and formula—start looking good when you're having problems. Some mothers can't imagine how they'll ever overcome their difficulties and achieve that positive, successful breastfeeding experience they dreamed of. No matter what you face, you need to remember that breastfeeding takes commitment and support. With determination and guidance, you can overcome any problem and find a way to give your baby your precious milk. Before you know it, you and your baby will be breastfeeding without a thought and without a care.

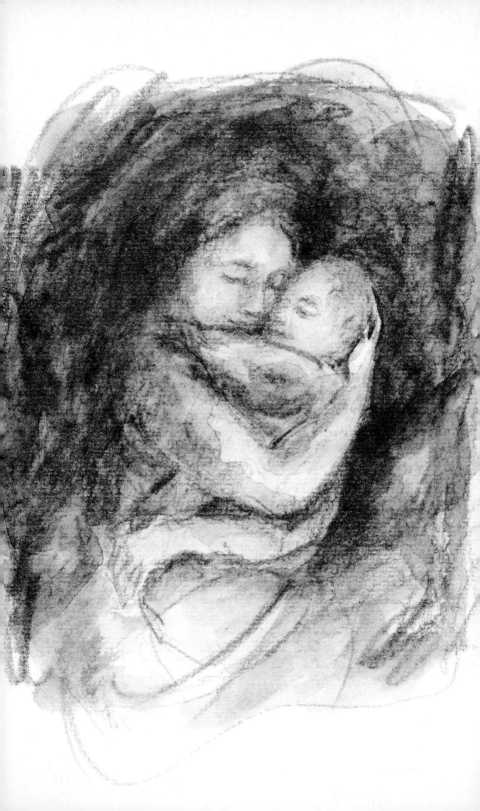

Chapter 7

DOWN THE ROAD

Three Months—and Going Strong

How wonderful! I guess you're looking forward to the months ahead, now that those first days and weeks of learning are behind you. I'm sure you hardly think about how your baby latches on to the breast now. He's very clever at getting on and off by himself and smiling up at you before he pops back on and has a little more. Now you can say with pride: "Breastfeeding—I can do that!" This is what breastfeeding is all about. Not only is it enjoyable, but it also gives you lots of opportunities to sit down, concentrate on your baby, and think about the nice things in life.

All the positive feedback I received while I was learning to breastfeed was great. My breastfeeding is fantastic now, and I can even talk on the phone and feed at the same time. Angie is twelve weeks old and putting on lots of weight. She was six and a half pounds at birth, and now she's twelve pounds. We have a lovely routine, and most nights her long sleep is four to five hours.

—Ruth

We were off camping last weekend. It was great fun, and Fin enjoyed two nights in a tent. At times like this, I'm really glad to be breastfeeding—rolling over and feeding is so easy! We even climbed one of the mountains with a few stops for feeds. Fin made it to the top with his dad. I stopped just before the top, as it was a bit windy and rocky! In those first few weeks, I would have never believed we could feed anytime, anywhere, in any situation. Now we are doing it! Pat, the child-health nurse, has helped us with expressing, and hopefully this will enable me to leave Fin with his dad for a few hours, so I can get back to some serious horse riding!

—Jill

I'm Growing Up, Mom!

Your darling little baby is about to take his first step into independent life. Instead of lying in your arms and looking at you during the feed, which had been his favorite pastime for the last three months, he now wants to see what's happening around him. Unfortunately, as he turns his head when he hears a voice or sound, he'll often forget to let go of your breast, and it'll stretch.

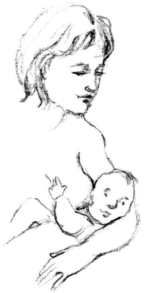

Your baby may also change his feeding habits. As time goes on, you'll find he requires a different number of feeds each day—three or four some days, twenty or more other days. He may shorten a feed from a half hour to five minutes, want a few more sucks twenty minutes later, then finish his feed ten minutes after that. It's a bit like how we adults drink and eat. You often don't have time to sit and leisurely enjoy a cup of coffee and a snack. Now that you're a busy mom, you make the coffee and snack, go do some chores, and come back now and then for a little more. You take lots of breaks, and your baby wants to do that now as well. He's simply learning about the grown-up way of eating and drinking.

Growth Spurts

Breastfed babies gain steady amounts of weight over the first ten to twelve weeks, then they level off as they become more active. But just when you think your baby's weight gain has slowed down, he'll be eager to feed more often, and his weight gain will climb once again. This often happens around three months, when babies have a growth spurt. The concept of "growth spurts" became popular in the 1970s, and with it came wonderful evidence for breastfeeding according to your baby's needs and not a forced schedule.

At this time, your baby will "tell" your breasts to make more milk for his larger appetite. He does this very easily by feeding, taking a break, and then going back to the breast for a quick top-off. He may suck for only a few minutes at the end, but that's enough to drain your breasts so they'll replace the milk faster and boost your supply. The more you drain your breasts, the faster they replace the milk.

During a growth spurt, your baby may feed frequently in the evenings. During the day you make about a half ounce of milk per hour, but in the evening you make twice as much. The extra production ensures you have enough milk for overnight and the next day. Also, by the evening, your well-drained breasts make high-fat milk full of extra calories for your baby's growth. If you start feeling frustrated by how often your baby feeds during this growth spurt, try to think instead about how plump and gorgeous he is because of your milk.

Things to Do

During a growth spurt, keep a diary for two days (see pages 72–73) in which you write:

✔ when your baby feeds
✔ whether he feeds on one or both breasts each feed
✔ whether he settles better when he has one or both breasts each feed
✔ how many wet and soiled diapers you have changed

Breastfeeding in Public

As more and more women formula-fed their babies throughout the twentieth century, breastfeeding disappeared from the cultural landscape. Breasts became nothing more than sexual symbols to most people, and breastfeeding in public became socially unacceptable. Even though breastfeeding is back to the forefront of baby care, two big issues remain: Society still sees breasts primarily in a sexual way, yet most people assume breastfeeding is instinctual and "easy" for women. This means many breastfeeding mothers worry about being as discreet as possible when feeding in public, yet they also feel pressured into pretending that they know what they're doing right from the start. For this reason, you probably didn't breastfeed in public very often or at all when you started breastfeeding and your baby wasn't latching easily.

Now that you and your baby are so good at it, hopefully you feel more confident about breastfeeding wherever and whenever you want to. Society's views will change as more mothers breastfeed in public—especially without feeling the need to hide in restrooms or under blankets. Over the last thirty years, mothers have fought for their right to breastfeed in public. To this day, we often hear news about a "storm in a bra cup" when women are asked not to breastfeed in such places as restaurants, theaters, government buildings, swimming pools, and on buses. The good news is: More and more laws have been enacted to protect mothers' and babies' rights in the past five to ten years. Many countries where breastfeeding in public was previously frowned upon now have antidiscrimination laws allowing women to breastfeed when and where they need to. Also, many states in the United States have laws making it illegal to harass a mother breastfeeding in public, even if the nipple is exposed during feeding. In Australia, many businesses, cafés, and restaurants now have stickers on their front doors letting visitors know breastfeeding is welcome there.

If you're still unsure or modest about feeding in public, ease into it. Practice at home in front of a mirror to see how little or how much you expose with different types of clothing. If it helps, wear clothes that cover your breast while you feed. As you'll see, if you pull up a loose shirt, it will cover the top of your breast, and your baby will cover the bottom. If your midriff is exposed, you can use a light wrap to cover it. Some mothers like to buy or make clothes with pleats or discreet openings or put their babies in slings when they go out. When you're ready for your first few feeds in public, you may feel more relaxed and confident if you're with relatives and friends who support breastfeeding and if you choose a quiet, comfortable place. In no time at all, you'll feel confident about feeding your baby anywhere.

Enjoying the Two of You Again

Having a baby is so wonderful—and time-consuming—that you may find that you need to be with him all the time, especially during the early months. At some point, though, it's important to make time to enjoy some of the things you and your partner used to do before your baby was born.

If leaving the baby with a sitter isn't feasible yet, you need to work around your baby's unpredictable evening needs to make the most of your precious time together. If you manage this time wisely, it can be a wonderful way to revitalize your relationship. For example, you and your partner most likely "divide and conquer," with one of you focusing on the baby and the other focusing on cooking or chores. Instead, try to find a way to do these activities together, such as feeding the baby in the kitchen so you can chat while your partner makes supper. Some evenings you may enjoy having dinner with family or friends, where there will be other willing arms to hold your baby. Then you can concentrate on eating and catching up with each other and your friends.

If you're able to go out for an evening without your baby, you need to plan ahead so you have enough expressed milk for the sitter to feed him. Breastfeed just before you leave so you don't become overfull and uncomfortable while you're out. It may be helpful to leave a piece of your clothing for the sitter to drape over his or her shoulder or around the bottle so your smell will encourage your baby to drink well even though you're not there.

Sexuality and Fertility

Sexuality is a key part of revitalizing your relationship after the baby arrives. Some breastfeeding women say they're less easily aroused, while others say their libidos are heightened; some prefer just to be cuddled and stroked, while others are interested in intercourse. (In addition to hormonal changes, most new mothers suffer from sleep deprivation, so sex is sometimes the last thing on their minds!) Talk to your partner about your feelings about sex, and find a way to meet both your needs.

While you breastfeed, a number of hormones control your sexuality and fertility. These include estrogen, oxytocin, and gonadotropin-releasing hormone (GnRH).

Estrogen

After your baby is born, your estrogen levels are low until just before your first ovulation, which will be delayed under certain breastfeeding conditions (see page 120), or which otherwise may occur as early as six weeks after your baby is born. The low levels of estrogen may affect your libido, as it's the hormone that makes you feel sexy and keeps your vagina lubricated.

Oxytocin

As explained in Chapter 1 (see page 3), oxytocin is released during love, labor, and lactation, and it makes you feel good. The calming effect from oxytocin at each feed may either lessen your need for intercourse or increase your sexual responsiveness.

When you have intercourse and oxytocin is released, your breasts will leak, so if tonight is the night:

- Feed and settle your baby first.
- Take a towel to bed to catch the flow.
- Use the milk flow as part of your enjoyment—breastmilk is good for adults to drink as well as for babies.
- Know that there will be plenty of milk still in your breasts if your baby wakes up.

Gonadotropin-Releasing Hormone (GnRH)

GnRH is the hormone that begins ovulation. Research suggests that regular nipple stimulation during breastfeeding leads to high levels of endorphins, which stop the release of GnRH and therefore suppress ovulation.[1] Under the right conditions, breastfeeding acts as a natural contraceptive. If suckling continues around the clock and your baby's interest in suckling is not affected by solids or the fairly constant use of a dummy (such as a pacifier), your GnRH level will remain low and ovulation is less likely to occur.

> Giving your baby a pacifier even for five minutes before or after each feed can reduce the natural contraceptive effect of breastfeeding. If you give the pacifier for five minutes at eight feeds, your breasts will miss out on forty minutes of stimulation every twenty-four hours. This may allow your GnRH level to increase, may cause you to ovulate, and may lead to pregnancy if you don't use some other form of contraception.

The Bellagio Consensus Conference in 1988 established that breastfeeding is 98.8 percent effective as a contraceptive if your baby is less than six months old and:

- You haven't had a menstrual period since the birth of your baby.
- Your baby wakes for feeds during the night.
- Your baby isn't having other liquids or solids.
- Your baby doesn't frequently suck on a dummy.[2]

If you don't meet one of the above criteria, you need to discuss the use of another contraceptive method with your caregiver. Barrier methods such as condoms or cervical caps will not affect your breastmilk supply, whereas oral contraceptives may have some effect on it.[3]

You *Can* Work and Breastfeed

Most women in the twenty-first century return to the paid workforce within weeks or months of their babies' births. Many of those women assume they can't breastfeed *and* work, and they think they need to wean their babies. In fact, there's often no need to wean. If you return to work, you can express and store your milk, which a care provider can bottle-feed to your baby. This maintains your supply, and it eliminates the need for your baby to have formula when you're not there to feed him from the breast. Returning to work and leaving your baby can be hard, but women who express and feed at the breast, even if for only a few feeds each day, often cope much more easily than those who wean. You'll discover how lovely it is to collect your baby after work and see the joy on his face as he nuzzles in to feed. The wonderful oxytocin will relax you, and the stresses of work will disappear.

Here's a glimpse of how your days might look once you return to work:
1. In the morning, you'll enjoy a little time together and a breastfeed.
2. During your morning snack break at work, you'll pump. Your baby's care provider will bottle-feed him the expressed milk you pumped yesterday.
3. After lunch, you take a break to express. Meanwhile, your baby will have a mid-afternoon bottle.
4. That beautiful, smiling, welcoming face will greet you, and you'll kick off your shoes, sit down, and enjoy a feed together again.
5. You'll spend the evening and overnight with lots of cuddling and feeds, making the most of the time you share.

Breastfeeding when you return to work will obviously take some organization. This will be easier if you talk to your partner and/or your baby's care provider, your employer, and your coworkers ahead of time. Whether your partner will stay home with the baby or you bring the baby to a daycare center or care provider's home, you'll need to discuss the details of storing and bottle-feeding your expressed milk (see pages 57–58). Make sure the care provider knows to feed according to your baby's needs and not a schedule. Be sure to send enough milk each day to cover your baby's normal intake.

> After a few days of pumping and sending expressed milk to daycare with Tony, I got a feel for the range he might drink in a day away from me. Then I always sent just a little more than I thought he'd need at his hungriest. I made sure I always had enough expressed milk stored up (by pumping once over the weekend) so that even if one day's expression was a little low, I'd have enough of a backup supply to cover the shortfall.
>
> —Christine

With your employer, discuss how you'll need time to express during the workday, hopefully without losing lunchtime or other breaks, and how you'll need a private, comfortable place to do this. You'll also need access to a refrigerator to store your milk during the day. If a refrigerator isn't available, you'll need to store your milk in an insulated cooler or container, which you'll need anyway to keep the milk cool while you travel home. If your employer is concerned about your productivity during this time, it may be helpful to point out that research has shown babies are healthier when their mothers continue breastfeeding when they return to work; therefore, breastfeeding mothers don't miss as much work caring for sick children.[3] The immune properties of your breastmilk are essential, especially if your baby's in a new environment at a daycare center or care provider's home. You may also find it helpful to know your legal rights regarding breastfeeding and pumping. If you live in a state or province where these rights are specifically protected by law, knowing that law (and reminding your employer of it) can prevent unnecessary hassle. For an up-to-date summary of breastfeeding laws in each U.S. state, visit La Leche League International's website (http://www.laleleague.org/Law/summary.html).

> When it was time to return to work, I made a commitment to continue breastfeeding. I learned to express, and Mark, who stays home full-time with Aisha, took control of bottles and the freezer. Returning to work those first few days was a tearful and traumatic time, particularly because going home and feeding Aisha at lunchtime didn't work out as I had planned. As the days went on, we quickly settled into a morning routine

of a feed, a pumping session, and Mark packing my bag with the pump and bottles for the day before I headed out the door. As you predicted, Aisha made up for the breast time in the evenings and overnights (sharing a bed with us—too easy!).

Mark's coordination of the whole process was integral to our success. He kept tabs on frozen supplies and always let me know how we were doing for the morning and afternoon milk he bottle-fed her. Our friends rightly rewarded him the title of "Best Breastfeeding Dad" at our farewell party when we later moved.

For my part, I just kept expressing and bringing home the supplies. My staff organized my schedule around morning and afternoon expressing breaks. Even though being around a breastfeeding mom was new to them, my colleagues' support was really important, though I must say I've never received so much performance feedback: "That's not as much as yesterday!" As an added touch, they put a sign on my door saying "Mother on Duty" so everyone knew what I was up to and when. To this day I laugh when I think of the number of callers who had no idea I was holding the phone with one hand and pumping with the other—a very efficient use of time! Support from my boss, himself a father of three, was equally important. In a lighter moment, he said when it came time to remodel our office, he'd ask the powers that be to put an extra power socket in each office for breast pumps!

When Aisha was fifteen weeks old, I had to go out of the country for a three-day conference while Mark and Aisha stayed home. I built up frozen supplies and headed off tearfully, wondering just how mad I was for leaving my family behind. The next three days were a blur of expressing—in airport bathroom stalls, on international flights, in restaurants, in the hotel, and in the specially prepared room at the conference. (They kindly papered the windows of an office to give me privacy!) Fairly emotional but proud of my success, I returned home to find Aisha doing just fine and Dad in control as usual.

At fourteen months, Aisha shows no sign of wanting to wean herself, as I hear some babies do at that age, and we're both happy to keep going. Mark still stays at home, and I'm down to one expression at work a day. It's definitely been one of the most satisfying and important things Mark and I have shared with our daughter.

—Sally

You're Pregnant Again!

Congratulations! Although some babies wean themselves from the breast during pregnancy, this doesn't need to be the end of your lovely breastfeeding relationship if you don't want it to be. Relatives, friends, and even health professionals may suggest it's best for you to wean. They may believe continuing to breastfeed increases the risk of miscarriage or affects the growth and development of the new baby, but no research supports this. Some people may express concern that continuing to breastfeed will tire you. However, you'll probably get plenty of rest if you continue to breastfeed because feeding gives you the perfect opportunity to sit or lie down frequently.

People may also mistakenly suggest your milk is of lower quality during pregnancy. During the early days of your pregnancy, the taste of your milk may change. It will taste a little salty, as it does when you ovulate and during your period. This saltiness makes some babies fussy, and they temporarily refuse to feed. If this happens, you'll need to give your baby milk you expressed before the pregnancy or, if your baby is old enough, other fluids or food until he's happy to breastfeed again. Also, the amount of milk you produce may decrease for a short time, but then your baby will want to feed more frequently, which will increase your supply.

When the new baby arrives, you can enjoy tandem-feeding (breastfeeding both your toddler and your new baby). Once again, family, friends, and even health professionals may be concerned, suggesting your new baby will miss out on the tremendous benefits of colostrum because your mature milk is already in. Rest assured that the same nutrients and antibodies found in colostrum will be released into your breasts as soon as you deliver the placenta. Both your new baby and your toddler will benefit.

Tandem-feeding may seem tricky at first, but many mothers have successfully done it. You may want to keep one breast for your new baby and the other for your toddler. Or you may prefer to feed your new baby first and then let your toddler have the remaining milk. Many mothers who have tandem-fed say that their children loved being at the breast together.

Things to Do

✔ Ask your local breastfeeding counselor or lactation consultant for booklets on breastfeeding throughout pregnancy and beyond. Share this information with any family or friends who are concerned about your decision.

✔ Talk to mothers who have tandem-fed. If you don't know any who have, your local breastfeeding counselor or lactation consultant may be able to put you in contact with a few of them.

And On to Weaning...

Weaning can be a bittersweet time for both you and your baby. You may decide to wean at any time. If at all possible, try not to do it until your baby is at least three months old, so he receives the important health advantages of human milk. Some mothers wean at six months, one year, two years, or beyond. It's your personal decision, and you and your baby will know when it's time. Be aware, however, that because breastmilk is so important for short- and long-term health, the American Academy of Pediatrics (AAP) recommends breastfeeding for at least one year and the World Health Organization (WHO) for two years. If a baby weans before one year (especially before six months), he will then need to be formula-fed, which may lead to a variety of health problems (see pages 9–10).

Solid Foods

The process of weaning begins when you give your baby other fluids or solid foods, even though it may be months or years until he has his last breastfeed. The AAP and the WHO advise mothers to not begin offering solids until babies are at least six months old. As your baby approaches six months or so, he'll show interest in adding chewable food to his breastmilk diet. When you notice him watching you eat or trying to take your spoon or food out of your hand, it may be time for him to begin solids.

Offer new foods slowly, introducing them every few days so you can watch for allergic reactions to a particular food. If you have a family history of food allergies, you may want to delay solid foods for even longer. Small amounts (a teaspoonful) of rice cereal, ripe banana, cooked sweet potato, or cooked pear are often suggested as first solids. Offer soft, mashed portions of your food instead of buying commercial baby foods. Prepackaged processed foods often have extra sugar and salt and aren't as healthy as home prepared food. Your baby will be used to the foods you eat at home because he's tasted them in your amniotic fluid and breastmilk. He'll also be open to many different tastes because the taste of your milk changes each day, depending on what you've eaten.[4]

Leisurely Weaning

Introducing solids is often the first step in the weaning process, but at some point your baby may gradually want fewer breastfeeds each day. This is known as leisurely weaning. Your baby may like to have only one or two feeds a day for as long as you're happy to offer them. Even with infrequent feeds, your breasts will continue to produce milk for weeks, months, or years. As you introduce solids and cut back on breastfeeding, your GnRH levels will rise, and ovulation will occur (see pages 120–121). If you aren't already using a backup method of contraception and you don't want to get pregnant, you'll need to use one now. If your caregiver prescribes a combined contraceptive pill, this will also help reduce the amount of milk your breasts make.

Leisurely weaning is best for your breasts and for your baby's physical and psychological health. As you scale back the frequency of feeds, your breasts sense the last feeds and increase the concentration of immune factors in your milk. This is very helpful as your baby begins to explore the world around him and comes in contact with more bacteria and viruses. You may want to express and freeze some of this milk as milk cubes, which your baby will love to have after weaning. You can either thaw them for drinking or partially thaw them for eating as a delicious icy mash.

We've all settled into our new home, and I thought I'd take a minute to write. After my four months of painful nipples, Catherine went on to feed until she weaned herself about three weeks ago when she was really ill. I thought she would have wanted that comfort, but she didn't. Anyway, she was sixteen months old, and we had already cut back to one feed a day. Chris said how great it was that I had kept going that long.

—Vicky

What If Your Child Doesn't Want to Wean?

Weaning is easiest when both you and your child feel it's time to move on. Some toddlers or preschoolers don't want to wean and are very upset if they can't feed, because they love these special times and the attention they receive while feeding. Mothers sometimes give the following reasons (sometimes even if they're gentle fibs) to help convince their children it's time to wean:

- A new baby is coming, and the milk will be for the baby because he can't eat big girl/boy foods like you can.
- Mommy's breasts (or nipples) are tired or sore.
- Mommy's milk is all gone.

Just after her second birthday, Rose is very understanding about my "sore breasts" and appears to be quite content to just cuddle and chat about her day before going to sleep. For the first time in her life, I have put her to bed without a breast-feed. It's making me very emotional, but I'm confident that the time is right and I'm doing what's best for her and myself. I still have ten precious cubes of expressed milk for the sweet child.

—Jo

Rapid Weaning

Natural, leisurely weaning is better for your breasts and your general health. There are no safe medications to stop your breasts from making milk, so if for some reason you have to wean very quickly, you need to let your breasts become overfull before you express. When breasts are overfull for any period of time, they stop making milk. The following are tips for the best way to manage this type of weaning.

- Once your breasts feel overfull and uncomfortable, express as much milk as you can. This is best done with an electric pump if you have access to one.
- You may need to express again after twelve to eighteen hours, and perhaps once more eighteen to twenty-four hours later. After that, the milk will be reabsorbed by your body.
- When you express, make sure you massage any lumpy areas so you don't get blocked ducts or mastitis.
- Feed the expressed milk to your baby at every other feed to prevent the constipation that often occurs with quick weaning to formula, or freeze it as milk cubes.
- Drink herbal remedies such as sage tea (one cup three or four times a day for three days) to reduce the amount of milk you make.
- Put cold packs, cold cabbage leaves, or jasmine flower compresses (the aroma of jasmine has been shown to affect milk production) on your breasts as often as necessary, and support them with a firm, comfortable bra.
- If you aren't already using a backup method of contraception and you don't want to get pregnant, you'll need to use one now. If your caregiver prescribes a combined contraceptive pill, this will also help reduce the amount of milk your breasts make.

After Weaning

It's normal to have a small amount of milk in your breasts for some weeks or months after the last feed. At first, your breasts may be much smaller than they were before pregnancy, and they may never completely return to their old form. But the fat will build up over the next twelve months, so even if they look and feel different, at least they'll be a little plump again!

You may be sad when you share that last feeding time together, but you'll always be glad for this special bond over the weeks, months, and years. As your baby moves into childhood and beyond, you'll find new things to share together that will be just as joyful as the times you spent breastfeeding.

EPILOGUE

So now you have traveled the breastfeeding road. I hope it's been a wonderful journey with your child and your partner. Your family and friends may have encouraged you and enjoyed the delights along the way, too. Like a new driver, you've no doubt had some challenging days, when staying on the road seemed difficult. But like that new driver, you found the courage and commitment to right your course and move ahead. Once you conquered the problems, you cruised along nicely.

If you travel the breastfeeding road again, you may find it easier to maneuver or you may need to find detours through new rough paths. However, your joyful memories of your last breastfeeding journey will make this next journey easier.

The pleasures along the paths of your developing child's life are a joy beyond words. Infancy and childhood pass all too soon. Just as you'd take time to stop and smell a beautiful rose during your daily travels, take time to treasure your child's cheeky grin and the pearls of wisdom that fall from her lips.

REFERENCES

Chapter 1

1. Lucas, A., and T. J. Cole. 1990. "Breast milk and neonatal necrotising enterocolitis." *Lancet* 336: 1519–23.
2. Oddy, W. 2001. "Breastfeeding protects against illness and infection in infants and children: a review of the evidence." *Breastfeeding Review* 9, no. 2: 11–18; Hanson, L. A., et al. 1988. "Breastfeeding protects against infections and allergy." *Breastfeeding Review* 1, no. 13: 19–22; and American Academy of Pediatrics Policy Statement. 1997. "Breastfeeding and the use of human milk." *Pediatrics* 100, no. 6: 1035–39.
3. FDA News. "FDA alerts public regarding recall of powdered infant formula." http://www.fda.gov/bbs/topics/NEWS/2002/NEW00849.html; and World Health Organization. "Joint FAO/WHO workshop on *Enterobacter sakazakii* and other microorganisms in powdered infant formula, Geneva, 2–5 February 2004." http://www.who.int/foodsafety/publications/micro/feb2004/en/.
4. Cox, S. G., and C. J. Turnbull. 1998. "Developing effective interactions to improve breastfeeding outcomes." *Breastfeeding Review* 6, no. 2: 11–22.

Chapter 2

1. Blair, P. S., P. Sidebotham, P. J. Berry, M. Evans, and P. J. Fleming. 2006. "Major epidemiological changes in sudden infant death syndrome: a 20-year population-based study in the UK." *Lancet* 367: 277–78.
2. Jamieson, L. 1994. "Getting it together." *Nursing Times* 90, no. 17: 68–69.
3. Bentley, M., L. Caulfield, S. Gross, et al. 1999. "Sources of influence on intention to breastfeed among African-American women at entry to WIC." *Journal of Human Lactation* 15, no. 1: 27–34; Saenz, R. 2000. "A lactation management rotation for family medicine residents." *Journal of Human Lactation* 16, no 4: 342–45; and Counsilman, J., E. Mackay, and R. Copeland. 1983. "Bivariate analysis of attitudes towards breast-feeding." *The Australian & New Zealand Journal of Obstetrics & Gynaecology*, no. 23: 208–15.

Chapter 3

1. Slater, A., V. Morison, and D. Rose. 1983. "Locus of habituation in the human newborn." *Perception* 12, no. 5: 593–98.
2. Lawrence, R. A., and R. M. Lawrence. 1999. *Breastfeeding: a guide to the medical profession.* St Louis: Mosby, 219–23.
3. Porter, R. H. 1998–99. "Olfaction and human kin recognition." *Genetica* 104, no. 3: 259–63.
4. Grammer, K., B. Fink, and N. Neave. 2005. "Human pheromones and sexual attraction." *European Journal of Obstetrics, Gynecology, and Reproductive Biology* 118, no. 2: 135–42.
5. Varendi, H., and R. H. Porter. 2001. "Breast odour as the only maternal stimulus elicits crawling towards the odour source." *Acta Paediatrica* 90, no. 4: 372–75; and Varendi, H., J. Porter, and J. Winberg. 1994. "Does the newborn baby find the nipple by smell?" *Lancet* 344: 989–90.
6. Mennella, J. A., A. Johnson, G. K. Beauchamp. 1995. "Garlic ingestion by pregnant women alters the odor of amniotic fluid." *Chemical Senses* 20, no. 2: 207–9; and Mennella, J. A., and Beauchamp, G. K. 1991. "Maternal diet alters the sensory qualities of human milk and the nursling's behaviour." *Pediatrics* 88, no. 4: 737–44.
7. Fifer, W. P., and C. M. Moon. 1994. "The role of mother's voice in the organization of brain function in the newborn." *Acta Paediatrica Supplement* 397: 86–93.

8. Matthiesen, A. S., A. B. Ransjo-Arvidson, E. Nissen, and K. Uvnäs-Moberg. 2001. "Postpartum maternal oxytocin release by newborns: effects of infant hand massage and sucking." *Birth* 28, no. 1: 13–19.

9. Bergman, N. J., L. L. Linley, and S. R. Fawcus. 2004. "Randomized controlled trial of skin-to-skin contact from birth versus conventional incubator for physiological stabilization in 1200- to 2199-gram newborns." *Acta Paediatrica* 93, no. 6: 779–85; and Bergman, N. "Kangaroo mother care." http://www.kangaroomothercare.com.

Chapter 4

1. Righard, L., and M. O. Alade. 1990. "Effect of delivery room routines on success of first breastfeed." *Lancet* 336: 1105–7.

2. Ebrahim, G. J. 1978. *Breast feeding: the biological option.* Macmillan Tropical Community Health Manuals.

Chapter 5

1. Ramsay, D. T., J. C. Kent, R. A. Owens, and P. E. Hartmann. 2004. "Ultrasound imaging of milk ejection in the breast of lactating women." *Pediatrics* 113, no. 2: 361–67.

2. Kent, J. C., L. R. Mitoulas, et al. 2006. "Volume and frequency of breastfeedings and fat content of breast milk throughout the day." *Pediatrics* 117, no. 3: e387–95.

3. McKenna, J. J. 2000. "Mother and infant co-sleeping with breastfeeding as adaptation not pathology: culture, infant sleep and SIDS." Australian lecture tour, sponsored by Capers Bookstore. (Notes available on request.)

4. American Academy of Pediatrics Task Force on Sudden Infant Death Syndrome. 2005. "The changing concept of sudden infant death syndrome: diagnostic coding shifts, controversies regarding the sleeping environment, and new variables to consider in reducing risk." *Pediatrics* 116, no. 5: 1245–55; International Lactation Consultant Association. 2005. "ILCA response to policy statement by AAP task force on SIDs." http://www.ilca.org/news/SIDSstatementresponse.php; and McKenna, J. J., and S. S. Mosko. 1994. "Sleep and arousal, synchrony and independence, among mothers and infants sleeping apart and together (same bed): an experiment in evolutionary medicine." *Acta Paediatrica Supplement* 397: 94–102.

5. Ponsonby, A. L., T. Dwyer, D. Couper, and J. Cochrane. 1998. "Association between use of a quilt and sudden infant death syndrome: case-control study." *British Medical Journal* 316: 195–96; and Scragg, R., E. A. Mitchell, B. J. Taylor, et al. 1993. "Bed sharing, smoking, and alcohol in the sudden infant death syndrome: New Zealand cot death study group." *British Medical Journal* 307: 1312–18.

Chapter 6

1. Joanna Briggs Institute. 2003. "The management of nipple pain and/or trauma associated with breastfeeding." *Best Practice* 7, no. 3.

2. Ramsay, D. T., J. C. Kent, R. A. Owens, and P. E. Hartmann. 2004. "Ultrasound imaging of milk ejection in the breast of lactating women." *Pediatrics* 113, no. 2: 361–67.

3. Noble, R. 1991. "Milk under the skin (milk blister): a simple problem causing other breast conditions." *Breastfeeding Review* 2, no. 3: 118–19; and Day, J. 2001. "Report of Australian Breastfeeding Association white spot study." Lactation Resource Centre *Topics in Breastfeeding*, Set 13.

4. Lawlor-Smith, L., and C. Lawlor-Smith. 1997. "Vasospasm of the nipple—a manifestation of Raynaud's phenomenon: case reports." *British Medical Journal* 314: 644–45; and L. Lawlor-Smith. 2003. "Nipple vasospasm: a preventable cause of breastfeeding failure." Proceedings from International Lactation Consultant Association Conference in Sydney: 529–33.

5. Mennella, J. A., A. Johnson, G. K. Beauchamp. 1995. "Garlic ingestion by pregnant women alters the odor of amniotic fluid." *Chemical Senses* 20, no. 2: 207–9.

6. Hale, T. W. 2006. *Medications and mothers' milk.* 12th edition. Texas: Hale Publishing.

7. Bowlby, J. 1977. "The making and breaking of affectional bonds." *British Journal of Psychiatry* 130: 421–31.

8. Barker, R. 1993. "The challenge of helping the crying baby." Lactation Resource Centre *Topics in Breastfeeding*, Set 5.

9. National Health and Medical Research Council. 1998. *Infant feeding guidelines for health workers*. Commonwealth of Australia: Australian Government Publishing Service, 41.

10. Ilett, K. F., T. W. Hale, et al. 2003. "Use of nicotine patches in breast-feeding mothers: transfer of nicotine and cotinine into human milk." *Clinical Pharmacology Therapeutics* 74, no. 6: 516–24.

11. Mennella, J. A., and G. K. Beauchamp. 1992. "The transfer of alcohol to human milk." *Breastfeeding Review* 2, no. 6: 286–90.

12. Mennella, J. A. 2002. "Alcohol use during lactation: the folklore versus the science" in *Current Issues in Clinical Lactation*, ed. K. G. Auerbach. Boston: Jones and Bartlett Publishers, 3–11.

Chapter 7

1. Short, R. V., S. Thapa, and M. Potts. 1988. "Breast feeding, birth spacing and their effect on child survival." *Breastfeeding Review* 1, no. 13: 23–27.

2. "Consensus statement: breastfeeding as a family planning method." 1988. *Lancet* 2: 1204.

3. Cohen, R., M. B. Mrtek, and R. G. Mrtek. 1995. "Comparison of maternal absenteeism and infant illness rates among breast-feeding and formula-feeding women in two corporations." *American Journal of Health Promotion* 10, no. 2: 148–53

4. Mennella, J. A., B. Turnbull, et al. 2005. "Infant feeding practices and early flavor experiences in Mexican infants: an intra-cultural study." *Journal of the American Dietetic Association* 105, no. 6: 908–15; and Mennella, J. A. 1995. "Mother's milk: a medium for early flavor experiences." *Journal of Human Lactation* 11, no. 1: 39–45.

FURTHER RESEARCH

Acolet, D., K. Sleath, and A. Whitelaw. 1989. "Oxygenation, heart rate and temperature in very low birthweight infants during skin-to-skin contact with their mothers." *Acta Paediatrica Scandinavica* 78, no. 2: 189–93.

Adcock, W., A. Burleigh, and J. Scott-Heads. 1988. "Hind milk as an effective topical application in nipple care in the post-partum period." [abstract] *Breastfeeding Review* 1, no. 13: 68.

Affonso, D., E. Bosque, V. Wahlberg, and J. Brady. 1993. "Reconciliation and healing for mothers through skin-to-skin contact provided in an American tertiary level intensive care nursery." *Neonatal Network* 12, no. 3: 25–32.

Affonso, D., V. Wahlberg, and B. Persson. 1988. "Exploration of mothers' reaction to the kangaroo method of prematurity care." *Neonatal Network* 7, no. 6: 43–51.

Amir, L. 2002. "Breastfeeding and Staphylococcus aureus: three case reports." *Breastfeeding Review* 10, no. 1: 5–8.

Anderson, G. C. 1989. "Skin to skin: kangaroo care in Western Europe." *American Journal of Nursing* 89, no. 5: 662–66.

———. 1993. "Current knowledge about skin-to-skin (kangaroo) care for preterm infants." *Breastfeeding Review* 2, no. 8: 364–73.

Anderson, G. C., E. Moore, J. Hepworth, and N. Bergman. 2003. "Early skin-to-skin contact for mothers and their healthy newborn infants." *Cochrane Review Library* Issue 4. Chichester, UK: John Wiley & Sons, Ltd.

Attrill, B. 2002. "Assumption of the maternal role: a developmental process." *Australian Journal of Midwifery* 15, no. 1: 21–25.

Auerbach, K. G. 1990. "The effect of nipple shields on maternal milk volume." *Journal of Obstetric, Gynecologic and Neonatal Nursing* 19, no. 5: 419–26.

Benson, S. 2001. "What is normal?: a study of normal breastfeeding dyads during the first sixty hours of life." *Breastfeeding Review* 9, no. 1: 27–32.

Bergman, N. "Kangaroo mother care." www.kangaroomothercare.com.

Bonner, W. N. 1989. *The natural history of seals*. Kent: Christopher Helm Publishers.

Bosque, E., et al. 1988. "Continuous physiological measures of kangaroo versus incubator care in a tertiary level nursery." [abstract] *Pediatric Research* 23, no. 4: 402.

Bystrova, K., A. M. Widstrom, A. S. Matthiesen, A. B. Ransjo-Arvidson, B. Welles-Nystrom, C. Wassberg, I. Vorontsov, K. Uvnäs-Moberg. 2003. "Skin-to-skin contact may reduce negative consequences of 'the stress of being born': a study on temperature in newborn infants, subjected to different ward routines in St. Petersburg." *Acta Paediatrica* 92, no. 3: 320–26.

Christensson, K., T. Cabera, E. Christensson, K. Uvnäs-Moberg, and J. Winberg. 1995. "Separation distress call in the human neonate in the absence of maternal body contact." *Acta Paediatrica* 84, no. 5: 468–73.

Christensson, K., C. Siles, L. Moreno, A. Belaustequi, P. De La Fuente, H. Lagercrantz, P. Puyol, and J. Winberg. 1992. "Temperature, metabolic adaptation and crying in healthy full-term newborns cared for skin to skin or in a cot." *Acta Paediatrica* 81: 488–93.

Cox, S. G. 1985. "Breastfeeding one side only each feed: a solution for the crying baby." *Nursing Mothers' Association of Australia Newsletter*, May: 3–5.

———. 1988. "Why are nipples a pain?" *Breastfeeding Review* 1, no. 13: 80–81.

———. 1988. "Why do some babies prefer only one breast at each feed?" *Breastfeeding Review* 1, no. 13: 85–86.

Cox, S. G., and C. J. Turnbull. 1994. "Choosing to breastfeed or bottle feed: an analysis of factors which influence choice." *Breastfeeding Review* 2, no.10: 459–64.

————. 2000. "Breastfeeding: a gradual return to mother's autonomy." *Breastfeeding Review* 8, no. 2: 11–22.

Daly, S. E., et al. 1992. "The determination of short-term breast volume changes and the rate of synthesis of human milk using computerized breast measurement." *Experimental Physiology* 77, no. 1: 79–87.

de Carvalho, M., S. Robertson, and M. H. Klaus. 1984. "Does the duration and frequency of early breastfeeding affect nipple pain?" *Birth* 11, no. 2: 81–84.

de Chateau, P., and B. Wiberg. 1977. "Long-term effect on mother-infant behaviour of extra contact during the first hour post partum." *Acta Paediatrica Scandinavica* 66: 145–51.

de Leeuw, R., et al. 1991. "Physiological effects of kangaroo care in very small preterm infants." *Biology of the Neonate* 59, no. 3: 149–55.

Drewett, R. F., and M. W. Woolridge. 1981. "Milk taken by babies from the first and second breast." *Physiology and Behavior* 26, no. 2: 237–39.

Evans, M., and J. Heads. 1995. "Mastitis: incidence, prevalence and costs." *Breastfeeding Review* 3, no. 2: 65–67.

Fetherston, C. 1995. "Breastfeeding twins: two onto one does go." *Breastfeeding Review* 3, no. 1: 34–35.

————. 2001. "Mastitis in lactating women: physiology or pathology?" *Breastfeeding Review* 9, no. 1: 5–12.

Gale, G., L. Franck, and C. Lund. 1993. "Skin to skin (kangaroo) holding of the intubated premature infant." *Neonatal Network* 12, no. 6: 49–56.

Gallagher, W. 1992. "Motherless child." *The Sciences* July/August.

Gray, L., L. Watt, and E. M. Blass. 2000. "Skin-to-skin contact is analgesic in healthy newborns." *Pediatrics* 105, no. 1: e14.

Hambraeus, L. 1988. "Nutritional components in human milk." *Breastfeeding Review* 1, no. 13: 91–95.

Hartmann, P. E., and J. C. Kent. 1988. "The subtlety of breastmilk." *Breastfeeding Review* 1, no. 13: 14–18.

Hartmann, P. E., and C. G. Prosser. 1986. "Physiological basis of longitudinal changes in human milk yield and composition." *Breastfeeding Review* 1, no. 8: 16–20.

Hofer, M. A. 1994. "Early relationships as regulators of infant physiology and behaviour." *Acta Paediatrica Supplement* 397: 9–18.

Howie, P. W., et al. 1987. "Protective effect of breast feeding against infection." *British Medical Journal* 300: 11–16.

Humenick, S. S. 1987. "The clinical significance of breastmilk maturation rates." *Birth* 14, no. 4: 174–81.

Joaquim, M. C., et al. 1985. "The advantages of human milk in the feeding of the premature infant." *Journal of Tropical Pediatrics* 31: 43–48.

Katcher, A. L., and M. G. Lanese. 1985. "Breast-feeding by employed mothers: a reasonable accommodation in the work place." *Breastfeeding Review* 1, no. 8: 31–37.

King, M. T. 1939. *The expectant mother and baby's first months.* London: Macmillan and Co.

Klaus, M. H. 1995. "[Commentary] the early hours and days of life: an opportune time." *Birth* 22, no. 4: 201–3

————. 1998. "Mother and infant: early emotional ties." *Pediatrics* 102, no. 5 supplement: 1244–46.

Klaus, M. H., R. Jerauld, N. C. Kreger, W. McAlpine, M. Steffa, and J. H. Kennel. 1972. "Maternal attachment: importance of the first post-partum days." *New England Journal of Medicine* 286, no. 9: 460–63.

Ludington-Hoe, S. 1999. "Birth-related fatigue in 34–36 week preterm neonates: rapid recovery with very early kangaroo (skin-to-skin) care." *Journal of Obstetric, Gynecologic and Neonatal Nursing* 28, no. 1: 94–103.

Macfarlane, A. 1975. "Olfaction in the development of social preference in the human neonate" in *Parent-infant interaction: CIBA foundation symposium new series* 33, ed. O. Porter and M. Connor. Elsevier, New York: 103–13.

Marmet, C., and E. Shell. 1984. "Training neonates to suck correctly." *MCN: The American Journal of Maternal/Child Nursing* 9, no. 6: 401–7.

McBride, M. C., and S. C. Danner. 1987. "Sucking disorders in neurologically impaired infants: assessment and facilitation of breastfeeding." *Clinics in Perinatology* 14, no. 1: 109–30.

Meier, P. and S. Wilks. 1987. "The bacteria in expressed mothers' milk." *MCN: The American Journal of Maternal/Child Nursing* 12, no. 6: 420–23.

Narayanan, I., K. Prakash, and V. V. Gujral. 1981. "The value of human milk in the prevention of infection in the high-risk low-birth-weight infant." *Journal of Pediatrics* 99, no. 3: 496–98.

Nemethy, M., and E. Clore. 1990. "Microwave heating of infant formula and breast milk." *Journal of Pediatric Health Care* 4, no. 3: 131–35.

Nicholson, W. 1986. "Cracked nipples in breast feeding mothers: a randomised trial of three methods of management." *Breastfeeding Review* 1, no. 9: 25–27.

Nissen, E., G. Lilja, A. S. Matthiesen, A. B. Ransjo-Arvidsson, K. Uvnäs-Moberg, and A. M. Widstrom. 1996. "Effects of maternal pethidine on infants' developing breast feeding behaviour." *Breastfeeding Review* 4, no. 2: 73–78.

Pardou, A., F. Serruys, F. Mascart-Lemone, et al. 1994. "Human milk banking: influence of storage processes and of bacterial contamination of some milk constituents." *Biology of the Neonate* 65: 302–9. (Abstract in 1994 *Breastfeeding Abstracts* 14, no. 2: 12.)

Porter, R. H., and J. Winberg. 1993. "Unique salience of maternal breast odors for newborn infants." *Neuroscience and Biobehavioral Review* 23, no. 3: 439–49.

Prodromidis, M., T. Field, R. Arendt, L. Singer, R. Yando, and D. Bendell. 1995. "Mothers touching newborns: a comparison of rooming-in versus minimal contact." *Birth* 22, no. 4: 196–200.

Quan, R., C. Yang, S. Rubenstein, N. J. Lewiston, D. K. Stevenson, and J. A. Kerner. 1994. "The effect of nutritional additives on anti-infective factors in human milk." *Clinical Pediatrics* 33: 325–28.

Ramsay, D. T., J. C. Kent, R. L. Hartmann. and P. E. Hartmann. 2005. "Anatomy of the lactating human breast redefined with ultrasound imaging." *Journal of Anatomy* 206: 525–34.

Read, L. C. 1988. "Milk derived epidermal growth factor (EGF): is it important to the suckled infant?" *Breastfeeding Review* no. 13: 33–34.

Rendle-Short, J., and M. Rendle-Short. 1966. *The father of child care: life of William Cadogan (1711–1797).* Bristol, UK: John Wright and Sons.

Rey, E. S., and H. G. Martinez. 1983. "*Manejo rationale de nino prematuro.*" Proceedings from the conference *i curso de medicina fetal y neonatal,* Bogota, Columbia. English translation presented by UNICEF on video.

Riordan, J. 1985. "The effectiveness of topical agents in reducing nipple soreness of breastfeeding mothers." *Journal of Human Lactation* 1, no. 3: 36–41.

Schaal, B., and L. Marlier. 1998. "Olfactory function in the human fetus: evidence from selective neonatal responsiveness to the odour of amniotic fluid." *Behavioral Neuroscience* 112, no. 6: 1438–49.

Shrivastav, P., K. George, N. Balasubramaniam, M. P. Jasper, M. Thomas, and A. S. Kanagasabhapathy. 1989. "Suppression of puerperal lactation using jasmine flowers." *Breastfeeding Review* 1, no. 14: 43–45.

Sigman, M., K. Burke, D. Swarner, and G. Shavlik. 1989. "Effects of microwaving human milk: changes in IgA content and bacterial count." *Journal of the American Dietetic Association* 89, no. 5: 690–92.

Stephens, J., and J. Kotowski. 1994. "The extrusion reflex: its relevance to early breastfeeding." *Breastfeeding Review* 2, no. 9: 418–22.

Stockdale, H. 2000. "Long-term expressing of breastmilk." *Breastfeeding Review* 8, no. 3: 19–22.

Uvnäs-Moberg, K., and M. Eriksson. 1996. "Breastfeeding: physiological, endocrine and behavioural adaptations caused by oxytocin and local neurogenic activity in the nipple and mammary gland." *Acta Paediatrica* 85, no. 5: 525–30.

Uvnäs-Moberg, K., G. Marchini, and J. Winberg. 1993. "Plasma cholecystokinin concentrations after breast feeding in healthy 4 day old infants." *Archives of Diseases in Childhood* 68: 46–48.

Varendi, H., K. Christensson, R. H. Porter, and J. Winberg. "Soothing effect of amniotic fluid smell in newborn infants." *Early Human Development* 51, no. 1: 47–55.

Varendi, H., and R. H. Porter. 2001. "Breast odour as the only maternal stimulus elicits crawling towards the odour source." *Acta Paediatrica* 90, no. 4: 372–75.

Varendi, H., R. H. Porter, and J. Winberg. 1994. "Does the newborn baby find the nipple by smell?" *Lancet* 344: 989–90.

———. 1996. "Attractiveness of amniotic fluid odor: evidence of prenatal olfactory learning?" *Acta Paediatrica* 85, no. 10: 1223–27.

Victora, C. G., D. P. Behague, F. C. Barros, M. T. Olinto, and E. Weiderpass. 1997. "Pacifier use and short breastfeeding duration: cause, consequence, or coincidence?" *Pediatrics* 99: 445–54.

Wahlberg, V. 1987. "Alternative care for premature infants: the kangaroo method—advantages, risks and ethical questions." *Neonatologica* 4: 362–67.

Weizman, Z., S. Alkrinawa, D. Goldfarb, and C. Bitran. 1993. "Efficacy of herbal tea preparation in infantile colic." *Journal of Pediatrics* 122, no. 4: 650–652.

Whitelaw, A., et al. 1988. "Skin to skin contact for very low birthweight babies and their mothers." *Archives of Disease in Childhood* 63: 1377–81.

Widstrom, A. M., W. Wahlberg, A. S. Matthiesen, et al. 1990. "Short-term effects of early suckling and touch of the nipple on maternal behaviour." *Early Human Development* 21, no. 3: 153–63.

Woolridge, M. W. 1986. "The 'anatomy' of infant sucking." *Midwifery* 2, no. 4: 164–71.

RECOMMENDED RESOURCES

Books

Chilton, Howard. *Baby on Board: Understanding What Your Baby Needs.* 2003. Finch Publishing.

Hale, Thomas. *Medications and Mothers' Milk.* Twelfth Edition. 2006. Hale Publishing.

Hanson, Lars A. *Immunobiology of Human Milk: How Breastfeeding Protects Babies.* 2004. Pharmasoft Publishing.

La Leche League. *The Womanly Art of Breastfeeding.* Seventh Edition. 2004. La Leche League Press.

Lothian, Judith, and Charlotte DeVries. *The Official Lamaze Guide: Giving Birth with Confidence.* 2005. Meadowbrook Press.

McKay, Pinky. *100 Ways to Calm the Crying.* 2002. Lothian Books.

McKay, Pinky. *Parenting by Heart.* 2001. Lothian Books.

Palmer, Gabrielle. *The Politics of Breastfeeding.* 1993. Pandora Press.

Sears, William and Martha. *The Attachment Parenting Book: A Commonsense Guide to Understanding and Nurturing Your Baby.* 2001. Little Brown.

Sears, William and Martha. *The Fussy Baby Book: Parenting Your High-Need Child From Birth to Age Five.* 1996. Little Brown.

Simkin, Penny, Janet Whalley, and Ann Keppler. *Pregnancy, Childbirth, and the Newborn.* 2001. Meadowbrook Press.

Spangler, Amy. *Breastfeeding: A Parent's Guide.* Seventh Edition. 2000. Amy's Babies Company.

Spangler, Amy. *Breastfeeding: Keep It Simple.* 2004. Amy's Babies Company.

Videos

Breastfeeding: Mom and I Can Do That. 2006. Sue Cox. Available from www.ibreastfeeding.com.

Mother and Baby…Getting It Right—Breastfeeding: Positioning and Attachment. 1997. Sue Cox for the Australian Breastfeeding Association (Tasmania Branch). Available from www.ibreastfeeding.com.

Mother and Baby…The First Week—What's Normal for Babies. 2003. Sue Cox for the Australian Breastfeeding Association (Tasmania Branch). Available from www.ibreastfeeding.com.

Hand Expressing and Cup Feeding. 2000. Wendy Nicholson for the Australian Breastfeeding Association. Available from Australian Breastfeeding Association: www.breastfeeding.asn.au.

A Premie Needs His Mother. Jane Morton. Available in English and Spanish from www.ibreastfeeding.com.

Follow Me Mum. 2005. Rebecca Glover. Available from www.ibreastfeeding.com.

Organizations

American Academy of Pediatrics (AAP)
141 Northwest Point Boulevard
Elk Grove Village, IL 60007-1098
Phone: 847-434-4000
Fax: 847-434-8000
Web: http://www.aap.org

Australian Breastfeeding Association
P.O. Box 4000
Glen Iris, Victoria 3146 Australia
Phone: +61 3 98850855
E-mail: info@breastfeeding.asn.au
Web: http://www.breastfeeding.asn.au/contact/general.html

Baby-Friendly USA
327 Quaker Meeting House Road E.
Sandwich, MA 02537
Phone: 508-888-8092
Fax: 508-888-8050
E-mail: Info@babyfriendlyusa.org
Web: http:www.babyfriendlyusa.org

Breastfeeding Committee for Canada
Box 65114
Toronto, Ontario M4K 3Z2 Canada
Fax: 416-465-8265
E-mail: bfc.can@sympatico.ca
Web: http://www.breastfeedingcanada.ca/

Centers for Disease Control and Prevention (CDC)
1600 Clifton Rd
Atlanta, GA 30333
Phone: 800-311-3435
E-mail: cdcinfo@cdc.gov
Web: http://www.cdc.gov/breastfeeding/

The Coalition for Improving Maternity Services (CIMS)
P.O. Box 2346
Ponte Vedra Beach, FL 32004
888-282-CIMS
Phone: 904-285-1613
Fax: 904-285-2120
Web: http://www.motherfriendly.org

Human Milk Banking Association of North America
1500 Sunday Drive, Suite 102
Raleigh, NC 27607
Phone: 919-787-5181
E-mail: Fkenan@firstpointresources.com
Web: http://www.hmbana.org/

Infant Feeding Action Coalition (INFACT) Canada
6 Trinity Square
Toronto, ON M5G 1B1 Canada
Phone: 416-595-9819
Fax: 416-591-9355
E-mail: info@infactcanada.ca
Web: http://www.infactcanada.ca/

International Lactation Consultant Association (ILCA)
1500 Sunday Drive, Suite 102
Raleigh, NC 27607
Phone: 919-861-5577
Fax: 919-787-4916
E-mail: info@ilca.org
Web: http://www.ilca.org/
To find an IBCLC: http://gotwww.net/ilca/

La Leche League International (LLLI)
1400 N. Meacham Road
Schaumburg, IL 60173-4808
Phone: 847-519-7730
E-mail: llli@llli.org
Web: http://www.lalecheleague.org/

La Leche League Canada
12050 Main St. W.
P.O. Box 700
Winchester, ON K0C 2K0 CANADA
Phone: 613-774-1842
Fax: 613-774-1840
E-mail: ofm@LLLC.ca
Web: http://www.lalecheleaguecanada.ca/

For contact information for La Leche League International organizations in other countries,
go to http://www.lalecheleague.org/WebIndex.html

Lamaze International
2025 M St. NW, Suite 300
Washington, DC 20036
800-368-4404
Web: http://www.lamaze.org

National Alliance for Breastfeeding Advocacy
Contact: Marsha Walker
254 Conant Rd
Weston, MA 02493
E-mail: Marshalact@aol.com

National Healthy Mothers, Healthy Babies Coalition
2001 N. Beauregard Street
12th Floor
Alexandria, VA 22311-1732
Phone: 703-837-4792
Fax: 703-684-3247
E-mail: info@hmhb.org
Web: http://www.hmhb.org/

United States Breastfeeding Committee (USBC)
2025 M Street, NW, Suite 800
Washington DC 20036
Phone: 202-367-1132
Fax: 202-367-2132
E-mail: info@usbreastfeeding.org
Web: http://www.usbreastfeeding.org/

Wellstart International
P.O. Box 80877
San Diego, CA 92138-0877
Phone: 619-295-5192
Breastfeeding Helpline: 619-295-5193
Fax: 619-574-8159
E-mail: info@wellstart.org
Web: http://www.wellstart.org/

World Alliance for Breastfeeding Action
PO Box 1200
10850 Penang, Malaysia
Phone: 604-658-4816
Fax: 604-657-2655
E-mail: waba@streamyx.com
Web: www.waba.org.my

INDEX

Also from Meadowbrook Press

100,000 Baby Names
This is the #1 baby name book, and is the most complete guide for helping you name your baby. It contains over 100,000 popular and unusual names from around the world. It also includes the most recently available top 100 names for girls and boys, as well as over 300 helpful lists of names to consider.

First-Year Baby Care
This is one of the leading baby-care books to guide you through your baby's first year. It contains complete information on the basics of baby care, including bathing, diapering, medical facts, and feeding your baby. Newly revised.

Feed Me! I'm Yours
Parents love this easy-to-use, economical guide to making baby food at home. More than 200 recipes cover everything a parent needs to know about teething foods, nutritious snacks, and quick, pleasing lunches. Now recently revised.

The Official Lamaze Guide
The first official guide to pregnancy and childbirth presenting the Lamaze method of natural childbirth, this book gives expectant mothers confidence in their ability to give birth free of unnecessary medical intervention, and provides detailed information for couples to deal with whatever issues arise.

Getting Organized for Your New Baby
This interactive book is loaded with practical info and tips on conception, prenatal health, childbirth preparation, baby gear, household management, financial planning, childcare, celebrations, and life with baby. It's newly revised with the latest, greatest knowledge about pregnancy and parenting—plus key facts and resources to help busy parents-to-be make decisions.

The Simple Guide to Having a Baby
The authors of the best-selling *Pregnancy, Childbirth, and the Newborn* have written a simple, just-the-facts guide to pregnancy and childbirth for expectant parents who want only the most important, down-to-earth how-to information on pregnancy, childbirth, and newborn care.

Pregnancy, Childbirth, and the Newborn
More complete and up-to-date than any other pregnancy guide, this remarkable book is the "bible" for childbirth educators. It includes a thorough treatment of pregnancy tests, complications, infections, and medications and detailed advice on creating a birth plan.

**We offer many more titles written to delight, inform, and entertain.
To order books with a credit card or browse our full
selection of titles, visit our website at:**

www.meadowbrookpress.com

Meadowbrook Press • 5451 Smetana Drive • Minnetonka, MN • 55343 • 1-800-338-2232
Contact us for quantity discounts.